A DENTAL PRACTITIONE!
SERIES EDITED BY DONALD D. DERRI

PREVENTIVE DENTISTRY

JOHN O. FORREST
F.D.S. R.C.S. (Eng.)

BRISTOL: JOHN WRIGHT & SONS LTD.
1976

ISBN 0 7236 0435 5

PRINTED IN GREAT BRITAIN BY HENRY LING LTD., A SUBSIDIARY OF JOHN WRIGHT & SONS LTD., AT THE DORSET PRESS, DORCHESTER

PREFACE

THERE must be very cogent reasons for yet another book on preventive dentistry. Every intending author should be asked, or should ask himself, why he is going to all that trouble? His reply ought to be: 'Because what I have to say hasn't been said before, or not in the way I want to say it.' I have been distressed (but not wholly surprised) at the present trend in many published works dealing with prevention. The attitude seems to be one of replacement of the dentist's traditional mechanical restorative role by mechanical and laboratory preventive devices and a 'philosophy' which bids to replace the patient's hitherto enormous expenditure on full mouth rehabilitation by enormous expenditure on a full 'preventive control programme'. We have a new (costly) terminology that has developed and there is talk of the ministrations of such exotic flowers as 'disease control therapists' or 'disease control receptionists'. The 'new' discovery of 'plaque' has been hailed as something like the first landing on the moon. It is rarely mentioned that dentists have been dealing with plaque and practising successful preventive dentistry throughout this century (and before), without the gimmickry, special gadgets, audiovisual rooms, high sounding terminology, and hence with very little expense to the patient except for cost of the dentist's time. The tools he used and should still use are dedication, care, continuing evaluation of his long-standing patients, and above all a burning enthusiasm and a belief in the value of his work. In the current enthusiasm for plaque control there seems to be some belief that careful scaling is no longer required!

The attempt here is to show what works successfully in practice—evaluated over 27 years—and above all what works simply, inexpensively and with a minimum of gimmickry and ballyhoo.

The author's sincere thanks are due to Mr. H. Colin Davis and Professor A. H. R. Rowe for reading the manuscript and offering helpful suggestions. I am grateful to Professor W. J. Tulley for his help with regard to aspects of preventive orthodontics in Chapter 6 and to Mr. Jeffrey Rose for the information given in the same chapter. I would like to thank Mrs. Eileen Jaffe for kindly providing the illustrations for *Fig.* 34 and Mr. David Boxall for *Figs.* 35, 36 and 37.

I should like to express my thanks to Dr. Donald Derrick who invited me to produce this Handbook and never became exasperated at missed deadlines, and to Mr. A. N. Boyd and Mr. G. A. Moore of John Wright & Sons Ltd who proved to be so helpful at the production stage.

Finally, I wish to pay a tribute to Dr. G. H. Leatherman for encouraging my fledgeling interest in real preventive dentistry all those years ago in the R.A.F.

June, 1975

J. O. F.

CONTENTS

v

FOREWORD

Maury Massler D.D.S., M.S., D.Sc.
Department of Restorative Dentistry, Tufts University, Boston, Massachusetts

IN this book the topic of *Preventive Dentistry* is approached in a very honest and practical fashion. It is written in a lucid and attractive style. This is a refreshing contrast to the heavily detailed textbooks which rest on our shelves as 'reference texts' but to which we seldom refer.

It should be read by every senior dental student as an introduction to the *modern* practice of dentistry. It should be read by their teachers, and quoted frequently to bring into focus the true objective of a dental education and practice—the *prevention* of oral and dental diseases concomitant with the surgical repair of these diseases when prevention fails, as so often occurs. The practising dentist (general practitioner and specialist), to whom this book is directed, should read it as a review of 'where we are and what we must do' in the art and science of *Preventive Dentistry*.

In making his excellent evaluation of the large number of articles on *Preventive Dentistry* to be found in almost every publication, Mr. Forrest saves us many hours of perusal of the current literature on prevention.

CHAPTER 1

THE TREND TO PREVENTIVE DENTISTRY

'ARE you good with your hands?' is the standard question all would-be entrants to dental schools have been asked ever since the beginning of formal training. It may be that the candidate's ability to demonstrate manual skills is still considered to be the most important attribute. For most of the history of dentistry this attitude has probably been correct because the profession was looked upon as wholly carrying out operations on patients, or as dental technicians with a professional background. For too long a period dental students were stigmatized by remarks such as, 'He couldn't do well enough in his pre-medical examination papers and so we've put him into dentistry because he has always been good at messing about making things in the carpentry class.' Of course this attitude has not been completely one-sided. Men with brilliant minds have regularly entered the profession and have been involved in the many remarkable advances made in our field. Yet how often has one heard (and still does), 'He's much too bright to go into general dental practice.' A further extension of this attitude is exemplified by the fact that often a really first-class dental technician has been persuaded to take the dental course, and many have actually done very good work indeed by the standards of the day. It cannot be maintained that this is a wholly satisfactory state of affairs for the profession. It is probable that the result of accepting the 'good with your hands' definition is that—

1. We have lost the services of those who did not consider themselves technically able or who did not care much for handicrafts.
2. The dental profession in all countries has concentrated on work which is almost wholly restorative.
3. This has led to the more remunerative aspects of dentistry being associated with the more complex aspects of reconstruction. The greater the destruction followed by technically involved replacement the more costly the work.
4. A large part of dentistry, other than the purely prosthetic, became identified with surgery, and hence the dentist was proud to call himself 'dental surgeon' and even jealously guarded his title of 'Mr.' rather than 'Dr.' (which was equated with the non-operating physician).

If we consider this last point which has recently led to much heated argument in the U.K. (is it fortuitous that it coincides with

1

the current interest in prevention?), one becomes aware of a few anomalies. Is the intending medical student who hopes to practise surgery asked at the outset if he is 'good with his hands'? Do surgeons come from the ranks of those 'not bright enough to become physicians'? Such questions would rightly be considered with scorn by all members of the medical profession, especially the surgeons!

We shall need the services of dentists with manual skills for a long time to come because of the enormous backlog of existing dental destruction of all kinds. But it must be obvious that the practice of conventional repair and reconstructive dentistry as we have known it will do little or nothing to slow down the increase in this destruction. Therefore it is necessary that encouragement, from recruitment upwards, is given to those who will devote time and effort to the prevention of dental disease. This is not as divisive as it sounds (save us from yet another 'specialty'). What is in fact happening today is that dental practice is taking the following form:

1. There are many dentists who believe wholly in prevention in all its forms, in research, teaching and lecturing to the profession and to the public, and clinically applying methods to put their convictions into practice.
2. Other dentists—at present the majority—feel that their training has equipped them to treat the considerable amount of existing dental disease, and will continue to do this to increasingly higher standards using more and more ancillary help.
3. Ideally an ever-growing number of dentists are combining the attitudes 1 and 2 above, and practise a modified approach by maintaining a preventive attitude to all the restorative and other forms of dentistry which are planned, and by simultaneously influencing the patient in a like manner.

Why preventive dentistry now?

There are those cynical individuals who assert that the current preventive dentistry vogue is almost wholly commercial and coincides with the sudden awareness in the last few years of the enormous potential market for preventive dentistry products of all kinds, for not only will there be large sales to dentists but also to the general public, and obviously this is, for a dental supply company, a very much more profitable new field. That this view is partly true must be evident from a study of the advertising in the dental journals where counts have shown a rise in the number of advertisements for preventive devices from almost zero about five years ago to roughly 50–60 per cent now.

This is not the entire reason or even the most important factor.

There are probably a number of coincidental causes for the present interest:

1. Although for years dentists were aware that much of their work, however expertly and carefully carried out, was liable to break down in many mouths, with recurrent caries or loss of abutments of complex and expensive bridgework through periodontal disease, they attributed this on the whole to faults in their materials or methods. That these faults—imperfect filling materials, difficulties in tooth preparation, etc.—existed is not denied, but when methods and materials became even more sophisticated and breakdown of work continued, some dentists became concerned that something more needed to be done. With the advent of the air turbine, cavity and tooth preparation became so simplified that tooth substance was removed in a wholesale (and sometimes indiscriminate) fashion. Much of this work has adhered to Black's principles of cavity preparation with extension for prevention, often taken to its limits of full coverage. And yet recurrent caries still occurred. The more treatment was given the more breakdown occurred, except in a fortunate few.

2. As modern dentistry became technically more sophisticated it also became more expensive and patients themselves complained about further extensive work which was required so soon after previous considerable expenditure.

3. The public was made aware of research into preventive aspects of dentistry often reported in news media with little basis on immediate fact (e.g. the furore over dextranase). Magazines and TV programmes featured preventive methods as less uncomfortable than conventional drilling. A demand for these methods has come from the public and this too has partly influenced dentists.

4. One's own experience with preventive dentistry lectures and courses indicates that the main interest has come from young dentists with about 5 years' practice history. At about this time their dissatisfaction with the results of their work reaches a peak and even if preventive methods had not existed they would have turned to some other alternative to the daily soul destroying method of earning a livelihood by 'amalgam pushing'.

We therefore have reached a position where quite a considerable number of dentists are keen to practise the preventive dentistry about which they have heard and read so much. Pressure is also being exerted by some members of the public and it is here at the point of change where the difficulties arise:

1. In the U.K. under the terms of the National Health Service there is no encouragement of preventive methods in dentistry. At least, this is the belief of the majority of dentists. It must, however, be a matter of disappointment that a dentist can receive

repeated fees for filling the same tooth at regular intervals but no fee for a topical fluoride.

2. The dentist is uncertain which of the many advertised products he should use. The claims may be conflicting. He is worried that some of the recommended materials and appliances are now very expensive.

3. There is uncertainty on how to explain the practice change to the patient.

4. An important question arises. If the amount of restorative work is cut down what happens to his income?

These doubts together with many others act as inhibiting factors and tend to delay the dentist's action in promoting the change. There is, too, the additional reason that the dentist is not yet convinced, because he has not seen it in action, that prevention really works. He is struggling with his basic training in 'scorched earth dentistry' which taught him only to cut out or destroy faulty areas.

Thus the following chapters will be devoted to resolving these doubts and explaining how the practice can make a successful change to prevention. But no text can inspire the same enthusiasm as the eventual chairside clinical evaluation of the effects of caring for health rather than treating already established disease.

THE PHILOSOPHY OF CHANGE TO PREVENTION IN THE DENTAL PRACTICE

It has been stated in the foregoing that many dentists are eager to make the change from purely repair dentistry to one which considers prevention as a first priority. It should be stressed to those who may still consider that it is possible to catch up with the growing dental disease problem by expanding the number of available dentists that the results of other countries have shown that this does not work. We may take as an example Sweden, where the problem of a surplus of dentists was becoming manifest (S.O.U. 1970) but still the rate of dental destruction continued to increase. Many authorities in other countries have, however come to realize that the so-called lack of dentists is not entirely responsible for the failure to halt the progression of dental disease. Indeed, one factor must be that as restorative dentistry becomes more highly developed treatment becomes restricted to fewer patients because of the increased time taken, and of course the considerable cost. As stated by Jacobson (1972), 'Highly developed dentistry creates a "vicious circle" of increasing need for dental treatment'. It must be concluded that on the whole our existing dental manpower has been misused and it becomes necessary to foster and encourage a change of attitude on the part of both the dentist and the patient.

THE ATTITUDE OF THE DENTIST

1. The dentist must be confident that preventive methods really work and must hence resist the constant temptation to follow his early basic training which conditions him to drill out the sticky fissure as a so-called 'preventive measure'.

2. Thus the essential factor in the prevention of caries is to *resist* drilling teeth unless this is completely unavoidable. The investigation of pits and fissures with a very sharp pointed probe followed by the burr where the probe *just* sticks is not good preventive dentistry. It often results in the patient possessing teeth which may be 'peppered' with small amalgam fillings and as Phillips (1965) has shown all fillings are susceptible to leakage. The incipient caries

Fig. 1. The first molars were filled with amalgam but subsequently topical fluorides were applied regularly. The remaining teeth are sound but the filled teeth require further attention.

in sticky pits and fissures (if indeed it *is* caries) will usually respond to repeated topical applications of fluoride solutions—and this is true whether the incipient breach of surface is on the proximal surface or on the occlusal. (*Figs.* 1–3.)

3. Prevention is a team undertaking. It cannot be carried out in isolation by a single member of that team. Everyone connected with the care of the patient must be aware of the necessity for working within a framework of promoting health first in all procedures carried out.

4. The dentist must believe, and show that he believes, that prevention really works. If he reveals uncertainty and lack of confidence he will be unable to influence his patients sufficiently for them to adopt the new attitude to dental health.

5

Fig. 2. The repaired part of the tooth is most vulnerable even if the restoration is better finished than here.

5. The whole practice, all the staff—ancillaries, secretary receptionist (and also technicians), must feel this same confidence radiating from the dentist. Many hygienists, for example, are regrettably trained as scaling technicians and have not had the opportunity at training school because of the shortness of the course to see the

Fig. 3. Pits and fissures treated with stannous fluoride become brown and hard. No drilling is necessary.

long-term effects of preventive methods. Therefore it is often necessary for the attitude of such hygienists to be changed to a less technically and more preventively-orientated one. We must also consider the patient to be a member of the dental team because of the importance of patient co-operation.

6. Prevention is a continuous process. It does not end with training of the patient at the first few visits but will continue throughout the practice life of the patient in the form of careful reappraisal of the patient's dental health control practice and the resulting oral state.

7. The dentist must be convinced that prevention does not consist of technical procedures. Neither is it a question of which fluoride, which fissure sealant or which kind of floss to use. This approach is a result of the reluctance to reject the mechanical approach bred into the dentist and also of the assumed desire of the patient (or Health Service) to receive something tangible and visible for the fee charged. It is the author's own belief that the present use of fissure sealants comes into this category. In a sense fissure sealants are currently for those who do not yet really believe in total preventive dentistry.

8. Preventive methods should be easy to carry out for both the dentist (or dental team) and, especially, for the patient.

9. Methods and techniques which are expensive either because of the time taken or because of the high cost of materials should not be considered as acceptable. This is a further argument against such materials as fissure sealants (*see* 7 *above*).

10. It is all too easy to believe that preventive dentistry is synonymous with caries prevention. In fact periodontal disease is responsible for a greater tooth loss and is often ignored until too late. And yet in the early stages gingivitis and periodontal disease are readily controlled and reversible.

11. Finally, and most important, prevention does not consist in placing one's patients indiscriminately on rigid plaque control programmes; it does not consist in sending them into an audiovisual room to look at pictures and posters. The conscience of the dentist should not be satisfied by presenting the patient with a bag of preventive aids containing toothbrush, dentifrice, floss, disclosing tablets, wood points, interspace brush and a pamphlet of instructions.

REFERENCES

Jacobson L. (1972) Training and utilization of dental personnel. *Oral Hygiene*. Copenhagen, Munksgaard p. 106.

Phillips R. W. (1965) Cavity varnishes and bases. *Dent. Clin. North Am.* March, 159–168.

Statens Offentliga Utredningar (1970). Swedish Dental Health Service: Expansion and Organization. *Sver. Tandläk Forb. Tidn.* **11**, 38.

CHAPTER 2

EXAMINATION, DIAGNOSIS AND TREATMENT PLANNING

WE should be aware of the different stages of prevention as relating to the approach to disease control:

1. Primary Prevention: Steps taken to ensure that disease does not occur.
2. Secondary Prevention: Detection of incipient disease and halting its progression by simple repair or remedial measures. Sometimes at this stage there may be 'reversal' to the normal (as in gingivitis).
3. Tertiary Prevention: Treatment of well established disease in order to minimize or eliminate the gross destructive effects, to restore healthy function and to resist further attacks of the disease process.

Dentists have in general started their disease control at stage 2 above. Their training equipped them to search carefully for early caries, and dealing with this was thought to be the best approach possible. The result was a mouth with numerous small fillings in the pits and fissures. At stage 3 above or later the presence of periodontal disease was noted but all too often this awareness came too late.

THE ORAL MUCOSA

Caries and periodontal disease are not the only disorders for which dentists should be searching. The dentist should be on the alert for more potentially serious diseases, especially of the oral mucosa. The report on *Oral Cancer in England and Wales* (Binnie et al., 1972) gives the number of deaths from intra-oral cancer as 60 per cent of registrations. This is largely put down to the predominance of late stage disease at the start of treatment. The authors question how adequately the dentist carries out his important function of early diagnosis. They imply that there is limitation of diagnosis by limitation of training.

The clinical examination has hitherto been a hard tissue examination: cavities are noted and often the drilling is started at the same visit. In order to overcome the 'conditioning' given to dentists during training the hard tissues should be examined *last*, the survey thus starting at the neck, where the lymph nodes are palpated for enlargement and hardening, and then lips, cheeks,

8

tongue, palate are viewed and if necessary palpated. Any abnormality should be carefully noted and the extent of any lesion should be measured and recorded.

THE PREVENTIVE APPROACH IN TREATMENT PLANNING

Before embarking on any course of restorative treatment, our first aim should be the maintenance or achievement of the oral health of the patient. At the same time we should also be concerned with the patient's general sense of wellbeing, which should if possible be improved. Our approach should therefore be along the following lines:

1. Establishment of communication between the dentist and patient.
2. History taking: general; dental.
3. Clinical examination.
4. Use of diagnostic aids.
5. Preliminary planning discussion with patient.
6. Initial preparation by a member of the dental team (and this to include personal care and training).
7. Reassessment.
8. Discussion of definitive plan.
9. Final treatment to be carried out (if any).

If we examine each of these points we can establish a set of conditions as a guide for relating dental treatment to each case as it presents.

1. *Communication*

It is necessary from the outset to listen to the patient who has originally presented with some idea of what she or he *wants*. This is the reason for coming to the dentist. It may be to restore an anterior incisor. It may not coincide with our own later estimate of the 'ideal' programme for this patient. It is also necessary for the dentist to introduce at this stage, i.e. as early as possible, the idea that the attitude of the practice is 'different'. It is one of prevention. This may be explained to the patient by a number of analogies, e.g. filling teeth without practising preventive methods is like putting new windows in a burning house.

2. *History Taking*

Usually taken in two parts: *General* (medical) history, past and present; *Dental* history, past and present.

It is logical to check on the patient's medical background first and having recorded any relevant facts to follow up with an enquiry as to past and present dental disorders and any treatment carried out. Sometimes it may be expedient to listen to the 'dental story' first, especially if the patient is attending because of pain or other emergency, and follow up with the medical history.

Any important aspects should be clearly marked and attention should be drawn on the 'work chart' to any special disorders requiring care. This is always effected in practice by sticking a self-adhesive red star to the top right of the chart—beside it the condition requiring caution, e.g. 'Rheumatic fever x years ago' (Fig. 4).

Complaints of oral pain are recorded as requiring urgent attention.

Fig. 4. Dental chart with warning signal (red) in top right corner. This indicates that special care is necessary because of some unusual condition, which is noted briefly on top of the chart but fully in the patient's medical history.

At this stage by listening to the patient it will be possible to discover personality problems, perhaps by hearing accounts of the patient's experiences with other (unnamed) dentists and, most important, an estimation of the 'dental I.Q.' can be made. This is a measure of the patient's ability to comprehend the facts about his dental condition and his keenness to be involved in any discussion of treatment planning.

3. Clinical Examination

This should be an examination of the whole person, not rows of teeth. It starts as the patient walks through the door and sits in the chair. Signs of weakness, nervousness, facial pallor, cyanosis of lips, exophthalmos, breathlessness etc. should be noted.

Following the history taking and discussion, the patient, who is comfortably seated, is asked to close the mouth (every patient automatically opens the mouth when approached by a dentist), and the face, head and neck are carefully inspected in the mouth-closed position, and any apparent abnormalities are recorded. Following this the patient is asked to open the lips keeping the teeth in occlusion and a careful inspection is made of the entire vestibular surface of the lips, cheek, gingivae and teeth. The patient is asked to open

a

b

Fig. 5. *a*, End of periodontal probe deep in pocket. *b*, Probe on outside of gum showing depth. The exact measurement can be read on the sliding handle (Svenska, James Rouse Ltd.).

and close the jaws in centric, and any deviation of the mandible in opening is noted. During closing movements of the mandible it is important to look for cuspal interference which may cause a slide in centric.

The mucosa of the lips, cheeks and palate are inspected with special attention for white patches, ulcerations or discolorations.

The tongue is examined for size, shape, patches or ulcers and the patient is asked to protrude the tongue and attention is paid to any deviation to one side and, if this is so, the cause is ascertained. The gingivae are examined: colour, form and texture are important. Crevices (or pockets) should be gently explored using a blunt probe, and especially useful are periodontal probes (of the Williams type) marked in millimetres. This should be introduced into the crevice or pocket with the probe tip and blade parallel to the long axis of the tooth. Another useful probe is the Svenska which has a measuring scale with which it is possible to read the pocket depths directly. (*Fig. 5.*)

It is doubtful whether there is ever any need to use a sharp explorer or probe. One's own early recollections of being instructed on examining for caries was being told to use a needle sharp probe which was 'leaned on' pretty heavily, and if it stuck then this was a 'cavity' requiring filling. The question of what constitutes a cavity or indeed caries attack is one which must exercise all the judgment of anyone wishing to practise preventive dentistry. Is the sticky fissure merely a deep enamel-lined cleft, or is there a breach of surface with loss of enamel, and dentine under attack? If this is taking place in the depth of a fissure, how does one know? If one uses a sharp probe to get down to the bottom of a fissure might it not break through the enamel at the base? What is going to be the consequence of leaving it all alone? It is difficult to make out any argument for the sharp pointed probe.

However, so-called 'sticky' areas should be noted on the patient's chart with the date of observation and they should be checked periodically for extension, or invasion of tooth substance.

4. *Radiography*

Other diagnostic aids should be used. It may be said that every new patient requires complete full mouth radiography of approximately 14 films. One of the great boons of today is the introduction of the OPG (orthopantomograph or panoramic radiography) (*Fig. 6*). This is not only valuable in the saving of time but total radiation is reduced, and of course it is very simple for the patient (especially children) as no films are placed in the mouth. An ideal initial radiographic examination today is one panoramic film and two bitewings. This gives an 80 per cent reduction on the radiation effect of a 14 film full mouth study. In the standard intra-oral film examination the use of long cone techniques as much as possible will give more accurate images (*Fig. 7*). The use of No. 3 (long) bitewing films with built in bite tabs combined with long cone on the tube gives a simple method of achieving coverage of many posterior teeth with accurate technique. The use of XCP bitewing and other holders (which many patients dislike) is not necessary in this method.

At this stage the dentist should have a good idea what the patient's 'needs' are from the point of view of bringing the state of the mouth as close as possible to the ideals established by his professional training. It would be surprising if the patient's 'wants' coincided with the dentist's ideas of his 'needs'.

At the preliminary planning discussion there will be a further establishment of communication, and the dentist should explain to the patient the need for an initial course of training in a preventive approach combined with the health preparation of the mouth by himself or the hygienist. There is strong argument in favour of the

Fig. 6. A panoramic survey gives a considerable amount of information quickly and with low radiation dosage. Note the clear indication of the alveolar level.

early preparation of the mouth (i.e. scaling, plaque control, training in home care) being carried out by someone other than the dentist who will be concerned in any reconstruction techniques. In this way the important nature of the initial procedures is emphasised and also there is no temptation or pressure on the dentist to start his definitive restorations too early with often disastrous results. Indeed, in the obviously neglected cases with poor care and recurrent caries, or existing periodontal disease, the patient is told that treatment may not begin until there is a satisfactory outcome to this first stage.

At reassessment following a preliminary programme there may be considerable modifications made to any previous tentative plan. This will be based on the patient's demonstrated ability to cope with the care of the potentially restored mouth. If not, the type of treatment should be tailored to the ability and the interest which has been shown.

Also, as Young (1965) has stated: 'If the (dentist's) objectives are too far above the expectations of the patient, treatment may be

13

a

b

Fig. 7. *a*, Long cone on X-ray machine used with special XCP Holder to line up the beam accurately. When using bitewing films with tabs it is often not necessary to use special holders. *b*, The new Rinn cone is an improvement because it is shielded almost to the size of the standard X-ray film. Thus there is little exposure of unnecessary areas.

rejected entirely or fail if accepted. A prescribed course of periodontal therapy may be the "ideal" technical treatment for a patient with advanced periodontal disease . . . yet be unrealistic and unwise without proper motivation. In this instance, the alternative of extractions and complete dentures may well be "ideal" from the standpoint of optimum oral health to a specific human being.'

The dentist must also be conscious of another factor, that of his

14

own technical ability to carry out any planned treatment. He should otherwise consider referral of the patient to someone he considers to be more capable of carrying out a particular procedure. He may of course opt for a treatment plan which involves simpler procedures, meanwhile informing the patient of the more elaborate plan if this is appropriate to the patient's case.

Thus, in summary, we may say that a possible successful treatment plan will involve a compromise between the patient's 'wants', the patient's 'needs', the treatment possibilities assessed on the results of reviewing the patient's attitude to home care and initial preparation of the mouth, and the dentist's technical capabilities.

Any omission of consideration of these factors will 'neglect to provide beforehand against the occurrence of failure and the re-establishment of disease'.

REFERENCES

Binnie W. H., Cawson R. A., Hill G. B. and Soaper A. E. (1972) *Oral Cancer in England and Wales.* Studies on Medical and Population Subjects No. 23. London, H.M.S.O.

Young W. (1965) Motivating patients to accept preventive services. *Dent. Clin. North Am.* **9**, 523–533.

CHAPTER 3

DENTAL PLAQUE AND ITS CONTROL

IT is now generally recognized that dental plaque is involved in the pathogenicity of both caries and periodontal disease. The exact mechanism of periodontal disease progression in relation to plaque is the subject of much research work. There seems to be agreement among researchers that periodontal disease is associated with the presence of bacterial colonies on the surfaces above and in the gingival crevice initiating an inflammatory reaction due to the toxic products of organisms in the plaque; the action of endotoxins and host reactions to the antigens.

The still widely held view in respect of caries initiation is the action by micro-organisms in the plaque which is in intimate relationship with the tooth surface. These organisms act on sucrose products entering the plaque after carbohydrate ingestion, and form acids which at the critical pH level (below 5·5) bring about enamel dissolution. Our preventive efforts relative to caries involve increasing the acid solubility resistance of the tooth surface (by the use of fluorides), carbohydrate limitation, and plaque reduction, but when we consider our methods of prevention in relation to periodontal disease we find that we have as yet one measure only which has universal practical application—plaque removal.

Plaque formation does not take place haphazardly but in a reasonably orderly manner. A pellicle derived from the saliva or gingival fluid first forms on the teeth. This pellicle is a thin, clear cuticle and is composed mainly of glyco-proteins. Very soon after its formation, bacteria of the coccus type (streptococci largely) are attracted to the pellicle which has a 'sticky' surface, i.e. one which enables colonies of organisms to be anchored. These organisms divide and form colonies. Attachment of the micro-organisms is further enhanced by the production by the bacteria of dextrans as by-products of metabolic activity. Later other types of organisms are attracted to the mass and a dense mixed flora, now also containing filamentous forms, results.

The early form of plaque is said to be more cariogenic while the later form may be concerned in the initiation of periodontal disease.

It has been known for a long time that periodontal disease is largely preventable, and that in the early stages treatment can be very simple. With further progression of the disease, that is with increased destruction of the supporting tissues, there is need for

16

more involved therapy, but until quite a late stage success can be achieved in arresting the disease and retaining the teeth in good function. Periodontal care, however, is dependent for its continued success on awareness, diligence and constant reappraisal by the dentist and the patient.

We have reached a stage in caries control where it is possible to reduce substantially the caries attack and with some goodwill on all sides it is possible to visualize a not-too-distant time when dental decay is no longer the enormous problem that it has been to this day. And all this can seemingly be achieved with very little active co-operation on the part of the patient. If we are to control or treat periodontal disease however, very considerable help is required from the patient and without it treatment is nearly always likely to fail.

For many years dentists were taught the importance of thorough calculus and debris removal and its beneficial effects on the health of the gingiva. During one's own training the term 'dental plaque' had not come into use, but very good results were obtained with debris and calculus removal all those years ago, and long before. But a number of cases responded either very slowly or not at all. The therapy for these patients, as well as the very advanced cases where by rule of thumb any pocket of over 3 mm in depth was not considered treatable conservatively, was to carry out a gingivectomy procedure. Unfortunately, many of these cases relapsed postsurgically and one of the reasons for this (but not the only reason) was that the basic cause—bacteria—had not been evaluated and eliminated. The dentist and periodontist were not aware that bacterial plaque was frequently invisible and so they were too easily satisfied that oral hygiene procedures were being assiduously carried out. Therefore, the failures were often considered to be due to systemic factors and there followed a period of intense activity in which various hormones, male, female and other imagined deficiencies, were either applied topically or given parenterally.

Much research has been carried out, and continues, into the obviously potentially rewarding line of plaque prevention (by antibiotics and chemical methods)—e.g. the experimental use of chlorhexidine—but as yet there is no acceptable material available. Thus there is no periodontal equivalent at present to the use of fluoride compounds in various forms in caries prevention. The importance of this latter measure is that it offers the health services— at the practice, community and public health levels—opportunity for controlling disease to a large extent without putting responsibility on the patient. This we cannot achieve in relation to periodontal disease.

There is a vast difference between results of research using animals and subsequent application in humans. We can all remember the excitement aroused by dextranase, which was going to prevent plaque formation and hence subsequent plaque-mediated diseases. Many of us had requests from the public for dextranase *now*, coupled with complaints that we were 'behind the times' because it was not part of our armamentarium. Fortunately, long-term experience has taught the value of waiting for reasonable assessment of newspaper 'miracle treatments'. Most recent work has regrettably shown a lack of success with dextranase even as a plaque inhibitor. Just as public opinion polls—even five or six different ones operating simultaneously using the most up-to-date statistical methods and computers—can all give completely erroneous assessments of quite large samples (as in election forecasts), so too can the research worker, sometimes using much less sophisticated methods, err statistically. The reader is warned against being bemused by some papers which profess to be based on scientific methods but may be lacking in clinical observation and judgement.

Well documented and acceptable research studies, which have been amply confirmed (and in fact were a matter of general observation by most dentists), were carried out by Löe and Schiott (1970). They demonstrated that by keeping the teeth completely free from plaque inflammation of the gingivae could be prevented. Conversely, by ordering a cessation of tooth cleaning in their subjects, plaque was allowed to accumulate in the gingival crevice regions and gingivitis ensued.

Löe and others also demonstrated that if brushing was so effectively carried out that all plaque was removed, then recolonization did not take place appreciably until 48 hours had elapsed and therefore, in this instance, it was acceptable to brush every other day. As, however, this degree of cleanliness is an almost impossible attainment with nearly all our patients, one should concentrate on training them to a standard of plaque removal which is effective enough to allow once-a-day brushing.

Much of this and other work on plaque reverses some of our own previously held views. We have all for years told our patients to brush after meals, especially after taking sugary substances. However, if there were no plaque on the teeth before consuming the meal, there would be no matrix to hold the sugars and other substances in contact with the teeth. Thus if we could achieve effective complete plaque elimination by brushing and other accessory means, there is a strong argument for this being carried out *before* meals! But until we do achieve a satisfactory plaque control score, it is probably better to stick to the conventional method and ask the patient to remove not only plaque but also the potentially harmful sugar residue after meals.

18

a

b

c

Fig. 8. *a*, The gingivae are inflamed and bleeding in a teenage patient. *b*, The bacterial film and deposits are disclosed using Talbot's iodine, which is very dramatic. *c*, The improvement brought about by careful brushing.

DISCLOSING PLAQUE

Most patients are unaware of the bacterial film on the teeth and equate 'dirt' with discolorations of varying degrees. The dentist,

19

too, is often not aware that apparently clean-looking teeth have heavy deposits. It is essential to make these deposits visible:

1. To confirm to the patient the presence of a harmful film and hence facilitate instruction on its removal.
2. To enable the dentist or hygienist, during scaling and polishing procedures, to confirm that the tooth surfaces are free from all deposits.

It was the simple expedient of disclosing media which changed the direction of periodontal care, and hence we owe a debt to Dr. Sumter Arnim (1963) for his enthusiastic proselytising (*Figs.* 8, 9). Now this was a most unfortunate change for the patient, who was

Fig. 9. Disclosing solution is more acceptable than tablets. It may be applied with a cotton tip.

almost immediately burdened with the total responsibility of plaque removal, and thus the patient's workload doubled or trebled. But the results were very good indeed. It became possible to treat many cases of gingivitis at the bleeding stage often with nothing more than very careful training in the effective use of the toothbrush. We know, therefore, that the patient has a fundamental role to play in plaque removal, both in treatment and maintenance of the restored tissues. It is not sufficient, however, merely to tell the patient to carry out these procedures. When a patient has been accepted for treatment the dentist has a basic and never-ending responsibility in motivating and encouraging the patient's role in that dental care and this applies to all forms of dental treatment.

The desirable properties of a disclosing substance should be:

a. Ability to stain plaque selectively so that this will stand out from the cleaner portions of the teeth and surroundings.

20

b. Absence of prolonged retained staining of the rest of the oral structures—lips, cheeks, tongue.

c. Anterior tooth coloured fillings should not be adversely affected.

d. Taste must be acceptable.

e. No harmful effects on the mucous membrane, nor should there be a possibility of harm caused by accidental swallowing of the substance or from possible allergic reaction.

Some Disclosing Agents

Pink Disclosing Tablets

Dr. Sumter Arnim introduced what are termed in the U.S.A. 'disclosing wafers', which are in effect 'tablets' of erythrocin food dye—an acceptable food additive officially termed 'F.D.C. Red No. 3' (a 6 per cent solution in water). Examples of these commercially are given in Appendix 1. A cheap form of erythrocin liquid is Rayners Rose Pink food dye in 1 or 4 oz bottles.

Iodine Based Solutions

A formula is given in Appendix 1. The advantage of the iodine based solutions is that their effect is very dramatic. Plaque is stained deeply—brown or black—and the associated inflamed gingivae also show up as dark areas. It is then very easy to demonstrate the ill-effects of the plaque. The discoloration in fact disappears in a few minutes. This type of disclosing agent is excellent for clinical photography.

Another important advantage (hence lack of pressure selling by supply houses) is low cost. It can be made up by the local pharmacist. Two possible disadvantages are:

1. Some patients are allergic to iodine based products, and
2. Some find the taste objectionable.

Other Commercial Disclosing Agents

Every day brings a pamphlet describing a new disclosing solution or tablet.

After much experience of disclosing agents, the prescription or issue of disclosing *tablets* for chewing or sucking was abandoned many years ago. The indiscriminate staining of lips, cheek and tongue, which lasted for hours, was disliked by patients and they quickly discontinued the use of their tablets, often while still professing to be employing them. Similar objections apply to solutions for rinsing. Hence all acceptable disclosing agents are those which can be applied just to the areas to be checked—usually by a cotton tip.

The dentist should be able to evaluate all these new products by

21

trying out samples (on himself—this will also help his own plaque control!). A most effective solution would appear to be a recent one, Dis-Plaque (*Fig.* 10). It selectively stains varying thicknesses of plaque in different colours. The main objection to its use is its high cost.

Fig. 10. Differential staining showing various thicknesses and maturity of plaque ('Displaque'.).

THE PLAKLITE: Of all the plaque disclosing devices the Plaklite is the most interesting (*Fig.* 11). The apparatus consists of a small mains

Fig. 11 *a*

22

b

Fig. 11. a, The Plaklite. A mains connected lamp used with a fluorescein based solution. Two drops of fluorescein are swished around the teeth. *b,* The plaque absorbs the fluorescein and glows when the special light from the Plaklite is concentrated on it.

Fig. 12. a, Poor filling margins responsible for periodontal breakdown. *b,* Acceptable margins and embrasures.

23

operated lamp which gives a white light through a special dichroic filter. A bottle of a fluorescein based solution is supplied and two drops of this are introduced into the mouth and the patient is instructed to swish it in the saliva all around the mouth. The indicator fluid has a special affinity for plaque but is relatively invisible until the light makes it appear with a greenish yellow glow. The effect is startling and dramatic and may well be responsible for an added keenness to remove the offending glow.

MINIMIZING PLAQUE FORMATION

Having demonstrated the presence of plaque the dentist's responsibility is one of (a) removing it, (b) ensuring that the patient can

a

b

Fig. 13. Toothbrushing rendered more effective by the judicious removal of an interfering tooth. *b*, Note the improvement in gingival condition.

remove it and prevent its formation, and (c) so to order the anatomy of the mouth and teeth, where possible, to discourage bacterial growth and retention. Attention should therefore be paid to the following factors which favour plaque retention:

1. Filling overhangs (*Fig.* 12).
2. Open or poor contacts between teeth.
3. Unfavourable crown contours.
4. Cavities in teeth.
5. Gingival craters following destructive gingival disease.
6. High fraenum insertions interfering with brush placement.
7. Malaligned teeth making some areas difficult to reach (*Fig.* 13).
8. Ill-fitting dentures, orthodontic and other appliances which are neglected (*Fig.* 14).
9. Incomplete lip closure.
10. Excessive sucrose intake.

Fig. 14. Extra care is necessary when fixed orthodontic appliances are used. In this case insufficient emphasis was given to oral hygiene procedures.

The greatest trouble should be taken to facilitate and encourage effective toothbrushing which is our main method of attacking the plaque problem. This will be dealt with very fully in the following sections. All the disclosants discussed are a means to encourage effective brushing, and thus without the latter all disclosants would be a waste of time and money.

WATER IRRIGATION OUTFITS
(*Fig.* 15)

The use of these appliances which are expensive has very little justification in oral hygiene training. There is no question that they do not remove plaque and, although some of the manufacturers have modified their claims to that of apparently changing the character of the plaque (difficult to check), the trouble involved would not appear to warrant yet another chore for the patient. There is no doubt that these devices have led both dentists and patients to become complacent about leaving deep pockets because

a

b

Fig. 15. *a*, Plaque stained with Talbot's iodine before using pulsating water irrigation outfit (Water Pik). *b*, Plaque remaining after prolonged use of the outfits.

'pressure sprays will clean them out'. Regrettably this belief has often led to neglect of definitive treatment and occasionally acute abscess formation. It may be of interest to note that the Water Pik is no longer on the American Dental Association 'accepted list'. (Council on Dental Materials and Devices, 1974.)

It would take too long to give lists of all the gadgets and devices available. Some are described in Appendix 1. The dentist is advised to be wary and to give a prolonged trial to such appliances and materials, however highly recommended by salesmen. If everyone is still happy after one month he can possibly consider its further use.

POLISHING—A FUNDAMENTAL NECESSITY

One of the most important aspects of prevention is the provision of smooth well-polished surfaces which become plaque coated and stained less easily than rough or unpolished surfaces. This cannot be over-emphasized, and yet very few of the current textbooks on prevention even mention polishing.

One uses polishing techniques in the following situations:

1. Natural tooth surfaces.
2. The filled tooth, i.e. finishing the restoration.
3. Artificial dentures.

Some basic principles should be observed.

It is almost always necessary to use techniques and materials which avoid the production of heat. Both tooth substance and restorative materials will be adversely affected by overheating. Therefore, where possible slow speeds should be used and composition of rubber wheels, pastes, etc., should be checked to confirm that there are no ingredients which may be harmful to tooth surface or to filling materials (e.g. amalgams may be seriously affected by sulphur, which is contained in some rubber polishing discs).

Harsh polishing pastes such as pumice should not, in normal circumstances, be used on enamel surfaces, unless the severe scratching which results may be somewhat desirable as in etching techniques used in the currently developing methods of incisal tip rebuilding with materials such as Nuvafil, or in fissure sealing.

POLISHING METHODS
Armamentarium

Polishing instruments and materials.
Disclosing solutions.
For a list of the above *see* Appendix 1.

1. *Natural Tooth Surfaces*

Since well polished smooth enamel surfaces retain plaque less well than rough surfaces, it is necessary to polish all tooth surfaces after the removal of plaque and calculus which has been carried out as a routine prophylaxis or as part of a periodontal treatment. Many of the commercially available prophylaxis and polishing pastes are too abrasive, even flour of pumice, and will remove the more acid resistant surface layer or scratch it (Massler, 1969). It has been shown that more enamel abrasion may result from dentists' polishing than from toothbrush and dentifrice usage (Brasch et al., 1969). This would support those patients who complained that 'my teeth seem to get dirtier much quicker since I had them cleaned by the dentist'. It is also some sort of basis for another belief that scaling and polishing 'takes the enamel off'. Of course, all these complaints were, and still are, hotly denied as 'old wives' tales', but occasionally there is an element of truth, perhaps wrongly interpreted, in these beliefs.

The investigation above confirmed our own feelings which had led to the abandonment many years ago of the use of conventional pumice-containing polishing pastes. Additionally, motor driven polishing brushes are rarely used on enamel, the finishing polish being carried out with small webbed cups (of the Crescent type) held in a special angle polishing head or an old contra-angle hand-piece kept specially for this purpose.

Therefore, 'safe' polishing materials such as zirconium silicate (e.g. Zircate), tin oxide or even zinc oxide should be used. In the case of a scaling procedure which is prolonged over three or four visits and where, say, a quadrant is completed at each visit, neglect of polishing at the termination of each visit will allow plaque to accumulate as readily as before. In addition, the feel of well-polished teeth gives the patient a greater incentive to carry out home care procedures in order to keep the present smooth clean feeling for as long as possible.

The procedure for polishing the teeth therefore follows the pattern:

a. Very careful scaling, and if an ultrasonic unit is used much stain may be removed by judicious use of the tip. It should be remembered that deeply pitted stains are unlikely to be removed by a mechanical polishing method such as the motor driven brush and paste without reducing the surface of the surrounding enamel markedly.

b. Where possible, the proximal surfaces of the teeth gingival to the contact points are polished with strips. Anterior teeth are much easier to strip polish in this way and a medium width (4 mm) medium-coarse Moyco cuttlefish strip is the usual choice. It may be thought that a medium-coarse grit would be too abrasive but in fact after the first pull through the embrasure, when the grosser roughnesses of the surface are removed, the strip loses most of its grit and acts as a fine polisher. The 3M composite polishing strips which have different grits on each half may be used in those tight contact areas (through which the linen Moyco strip would pass with great difficulty) because the base of the 3M strip is of thin plastic. These strips may be passed through the embrasure under the contact point and if necessary a narrow strip (2·5 mm) may be used. In order to save time all the left proximal surfaces may be polished with the same strip which may be brought back and reversed to polish all the right proximal surfaces.

c. A disclosing solution is then applied to the teeth to be polished and the patient asked to rinse this away after a few seconds. Any obvious gross stains may be removed by hand instrumentation. The teeth are then polished by using a rubber cup loaded with zirconium silicate paste (or powder, made up to a paste with water) running at fairly low speed. All surfaces are polished and the edges of the cup introduced into the embrasures to polish the proximal surfaces as well as possible. The occlusal surfaces should not be forgotten.

d. A final polish (e.g. at termination of treatment in the adult) should include the use of a fluoride-containing polishing paste (such as zirconium silicate treatment paste), a disclosing solution is again used and any residual stains are repolished. The patient is asked to see the result of using a disclosing solution on clean teeth and then to run his tongue over the surfaces. 'This is your target from now on', he is told.

2. Finishing and Polishing the Restoration

Only cast gold restorations have the edge strength to cover enamel margins in thin layers without the risk of the restoration margins fracturing and leaving either the tooth-filling junction exposed or, worse, bare enamel rods. Thus restorations of the more brittle materials, amalgams, silicates, composites, should be inserted in cavities in which no enamel bevel has been prepared, in order to avoid the risk of bare enamel rods without their 30 microns or so of acid resistant enamel surface being attacked by recurrent caries.

Amalgam

It used to be considered undesirable to burnish the surface and margins of freshly inserted amalgam because this was said to weaken the margins. Recent work has indicated that burnishing may be acceptable as it has been shown that it decreased the mercury content and the porosity at the margins (Kanai, 1966). The better the carving and finishing at the insertion stage the less grinding and trimming (with the risk of overheating) at the later polishing stage.

Therefore the occlusal surface should be carved (some dentists use

29

a sharp scalpel), and burnished if desired. The surface is then wiped with a dry cotton bud to remove any free mercury.

If the amalgam filling involves the proximal (mesial or distal) surface this should be dealt with first. After removal of the matrix band and wedge, the proximal gingival margins are stroked with the side of a curved probe from buccal and lingual aspects to remove any excess filling or slight irregularities. Following this, a narrow (2·5 mm) extra-fine grit Moyco polishing strip is passed through the embrasure under the contact point (and if this cannot be passed there is going to be an 'embrasure problem' as described in the chapter on preventive aspects of restorative dentistry) and the strip is pulled buccolingually along the gingival margin to smooth this off while the amalgam is still reasonably soft. In this way one of the commonest dentist-associated causes of localized periodontal breakdown—the filling overhang—is avoided. Care must be taken, of course, not to interfere with the form of the contact areas between the teeth, provided that they are satisfactory.

Finishing and polishing is carried out after 48 hours and the surface is smoothed with finishing burrs or stones run slowly in the handpiece. Fine cuttle or sandpaper discs may be used, run wet if possible, followed by special amalgam polishing cones (Dedeco).

The filling should then be polished (together with the contiguous enamel surface) with mildly abrasive pastes and preferably there should be a final polish of the restored surface, especially the margins, with a fluoride containing paste and this may effect replacement of any fluoride which may have been removed during the filling procedure (Horowitz and Lucye, 1966).

Gold Inlays

Usually these will have been polished in the laboratory and should require no finishing or polishing in the mouth. All margins should be carefully burnished, however, and if possible the inlay should be cemented with a fluoride-containing cement, e.g. Fluorothin (S.S.W.) or Poly F (De Trey). At the following visit the margins should be gently polished with a zirconium silicate fluoride paste in a rubber cup.

Anterior Fillings

Whether these are composite, silicate or direct acrylic fillings, the main hazard is the same. Any overhangs at or below the gingival margin may be undetectable and these have been a frequent cause of localized gingival inflammation. It is therefore important to wedge the proximal areas very carefully after insertion of the material and subsequently to seek out any excess with a probe. A very fine diamond tip should be reserved for the purpose of clearing this excess. Messing and Ray (1972) recommended the use of sharp scalpels to shape off the excess composite. Fine polishing of composite fillings is difficult. The main surface is best left undisturbed with 'cellulose acetate strip finish'. Should this not be possible, smooth carbide stones are followed by 3M composite finishing discs—first the medium grit, followed by the fine. A fine rubber polishing wheel is also marketed for finishing these fillings.

3. *Removable Dentures*

The polishing of dentures is, of course, less immediately fraught with danger to other structures because this is carried out in the dental laboratory. The following is a summary of the more important aspects of denture polishing as it relates to tissue care:

a. The non-fitting surface should be polished to a very high gloss, and in the case of acrylic dentures care must be taken at all times in order not to overheat the material.

b. The fitting surface of acrylic dentures should have all the roughness and indentations removed and the surface should be polished to a reasonable smoothness. There should be no 'pimples' or excrescences in the surface as these will irritate the mucosa during the slight movement all dentures make under stress. Neither should there be any acute depressions which may collect plaque or other accumulation or organisms.

c. All sharp points including the dreaded 'collets' should be removed. These points variously can damage tongue, cheek and the gingiva relating to the region of the pointed denture base of clasps. The inside of clasps should be highly polished and the patient should have a separate careful demonstration of clasp polishing as part of home care routine.

Fixed Bridgework

This should of course be polished before final insertion. Any subsequent polishing would require the same attention as that noted for inlays.

It is therefore to be hoped that there has been adequate demonstration here that careful polishing is not just an extra that may or may not be thrown in 'if there is time', but is an important part of all our restorative and preventive procedures.

THE TOOTHBRUSH AND ITS USE

There is a multitude of different shapes, textures, sizes and patterns of toothbrushes available to the public. Most of these brushes, according to the buyer, were recommended by dentists. There are long head, short head, soft badger, all grades of hardness of natural bristle and similarly with plastic fibres. Some brushes seem to be quite inappropriate for tooth cleaning, others would appear to be not only ineffective but harmful. How does it happen that all these have claims to dentists' recommendation?

The reasons for the great toothbrush mix-up are many, but have never been adequately discussed in professional circles.

1. Toothbrush design and construction has changed over the years, but, in spite of this, many dentists have remained 'faithful' to their original concepts.
2. Our attitude to 'cleaning' has changed. We consider attention to plaque and gingivae more important than removal of food debris, and enamel polishing or 'whitening'.

The Nylon bristle fallacy

Many dentists still believe and staunchly defend their long-held view that *nylon bristle* is harmful and that the use of natural bristle is essential. At the present time this concept is erroneous and is a relic of a genuinely held concern about the quality of nylon a quarter of a century ago. (*Fig.* 16.)

If it were possible to observe the brushing pattern of a large number of people (as was the author's experience with adult volunteers for a toothbrushing test) a surprising number of important facts come to light.

1. Most people wet the brush under a running cold tap before loading with dentifrice.
2. Brushing goes on until the toothpaste has formed so much foam in the mouth that it then becomes necessary to spit and rinse.

At this point, however, at which little has been achieved in brushing around all the teeth, most brushers do not continue brushing after this initial rinsing of the mouth. Few ever reload the brush and start again. However, a high percentage constantly wetted the brush at short intervals during brushing. The effect of the initial and/or continuous brush wetting action is to make natural bristles soft and soggy. For this reason the majority of toothbrushes sold in this country were of the 'hard' or 'extra hard' type. But during the days before nylon, the extra hard brush became, after its soaking something like a soft or soft medium.

When nylon bristled brushes were developed initially, the manufacturers, of course, followed the same hardness formula as was apparently desired by the mass of the population. But man-made fibre was much less moisture absorbent and therefore when wetted as usual by the brusher it did *not* soften but remained hard, or extra-hard. The gingivae (and even enamel) were often damaged and at that time nylon bristles acquired a disrepute. Of course, this should have been referred only to the hardness of the brush.

Natural bristles
Natural hairs

Artificial filaments
(Nylon, Perlon, Dorlon or Polyurethane)

Cannot be
rounded off

Can be
rounded off

Cortex

Smooth, tube
and pore-free
surface

Porous, rough,
scaly surface
with organic
residues

Medulla:
favourable
nutrient
base for
micro-
organisms

No medullary
canal

Hygroscopic property
leads to softening
of the bristles and
loss in elasticity.
Risk of breakage
under heavy strain

Moisture absorption
below 1%. High dimensional
stability and rubbing
resistance. Indifferent to
chemicals

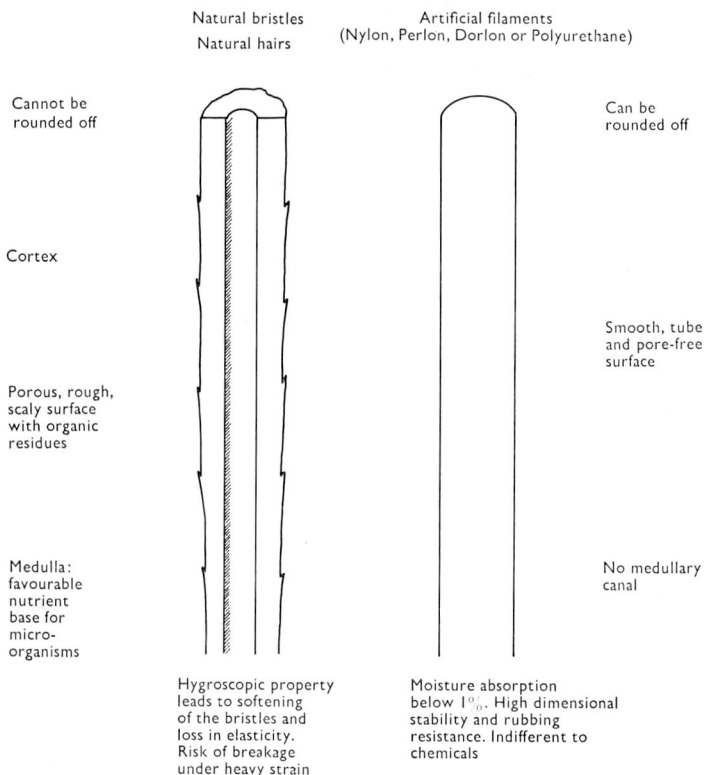

Fig. 16. Comparison between natural and artificial toothbrush
filaments. (*From Riethe*, 1974).

Eventually multitufted plastic filaments, which did not require
softening, were introduced and are superior to natural bristle for
the following reasons:

1. Plastic bristles can be quality and size controlled to very fine
   limits. We can make what we want to precise measurements.
2. Plastic bristles are potentially cleaner than natural bristles as
   they do not absorb fluids and organisms as readily.
3. Natural bristles take longer to dry than the plastic. Thus, if a
   dry brush is required a twice-daily brusher needs at least two
   brushes.

In view of the foregoing it is interesting to note that there are
strongly supported campaigns in Germany and France to forbid the
manufacture and sale of 'natural' bristle toothbrushes.

The Fallacy of the Soft Badger Brush

This was (and still is, surprisingly) recommended by dentists to patients who complained that 'brushing makes my gums bleed'. The badger brush is recommended to 'prevent further traumatizing of the gingivae'. The gingivae rarely bleed with the badger brush because its so gentle action achieves nothing at all. This actually fits in well with the brushing philosophy of most of the population (until now) who brush as a built-in reflex—part of one's cleanliness habits. No account is taken of whether anything is achieved in the way of plaque control: the aim is to do their 'daily duty' and to feel the 'fresh peppermint taste'.

If the patient's gums bleed when brushing, then one should find out why. If the reason is gingivitis associated with plaque (as it usually is) then careful training in brushing is necessary with the appropriate brush ('medium' could be used—*see later*) and the patient told to brush in spite of the bleeding. This will get better if particular attention is paid to brushing these inflamed areas.

The Fallacy of the Round-ended Filaments

Many toothbrush manufacturers (and also dentist researchers) show enlarged photographs of plastic bristles accompanied by a frightening story of how the simply cut bristles have roughened ends which will damage the teeth and gums, whereas the recommended rounding off of the ends is safer and healthier. (Sometimes this is called 'rondating', a term used by one manufacturer.)

If the dentist considers this to be of significance he should specify rounded end bristle brushes. It would, however, be of great interest if he could substantiate this belief by demonstrating actual damage caused by non-rounding off. The truth is that all non-rounded bristles become smoothed very quickly in use. This is similar to the use of a new comb, the teeth of which often feel very rough and scratchy on the scalp on first use, but subsequently are quite smooth (and the scalp is probably more sensitive than the gingiva).

The Choice of Toothbrush

Desirable qualities:

1. Man made (controllable) filaments—generally 0·007–0·011in.
2. Therefore medium or medium soft.
3. Short head (about 1 in)—straight handled—about 6 in.
4. Straight trim.
5. Multitufted.
6. But all the above qualities are relatively insignificant in relation to the essential quality—to be able to remove plaque from the teeth.

The type found to be most satisfactory is a multi-tufted plastic filament brush. Here many fine filaments are packed closely in each tuft and the latter are placed close together so that good coverage of the tooth surface and embrasures is afforded.

Multituft brushes may be—

Soft medium	or	Medium
Softex, Sensodyne, Py-co-pay		Wisdom multituft extra
Oral B 30. Oral B 40.		Gibbs short-head
Oral B sulcus brush. Dental H		

For the generally taught 'roll' brushing technique the Wisdom Multituft seems to be satisfactory and acceptable to the patient. For vibratory brushing techniques (such as is recommended in the Bass method) the Softex brush is more satisfactory. As the bristles are meant to vibrate in the gingival crevice the dentist may feel that smooth end bristles are essential. In fact, most of the larger manufacturers round off the end of the brushes anyway. The now frequently recommended brushes such as Oral B 40 or Softex have bristle diameters of 0·007 in. There is some difficulty in encouraging general and continual use of brushes such as these because patients do not like the 'too soft' feel of these brushes. They will, however, continue uncomplainingly with brushes where the bristles are slightly firmer—0·009–0·011 in. It would seem to be wasted effort to teach methods which involve the use of brushes which we recommend, but which the patients abandon. The Gibbs short-head and the Wisdom Multituft would appear to be readily accepted.

Automatic Brushes

Experience of these brushes from the earliest days of their development leads to the conclusion that only continuously powered or rechargeable brushes are really acceptable. Brushes with conventional replaceable batteries suffer from the disadvantage of an immediate lessening of torque from the first day of use.

All the powered brushes which are acceptable in themselves have quite small heads with multitufted filament bristles.

The potential for damage to the tooth substance or gingivae by powered brushes, a point sometimes brought up by dentists, is limited by the fact that no powered brush can exert the same pressure which can be demonstrated by the healthy-limbed manual brusher. The automatic brush would stall before excessive pressure can be exerted. However, in spite of the advertisers' claims, owners of automatic brushes must be carefully taught how to use them effectively. There is no easy way, even with these brushes. The advantage of the powered brush is that it is easier for the less manually dextrous to achieve some sort of result and once reasonable skill is acquired there is a saving in time over manual brushing. The potential disadvantage of these appliances is that the patient can be lulled into believing that all that has to be done is to purchase one of these and everything will be done for him! There would appear to be little difference in effect between automatic brushes which have arc oscillations, reciprocal horizontal movement or a combination of both.

Manual v. Automatic Brushing

All patients where possible should be taught initially an effective plaque removal technique with the manual brush. If the patient is manually incapable (or incapacitated) or even too lazy to spend enough time and effort, then an automatic brush may be recommended and demonstrated. Some of those who are able to brush satisfactorily with a manual brush may want to use an automatic. It is just as important in these cases to go over again the patient's technique with the new brush.

TOOTHBRUSHING METHODS

Although it would be a desirable goal, it is not possible to achieve 100 per cent plaque removal in any but the exceptional patient. We may try very hard to teach various techniques and follow this up with floss instruction and the use of interdental cleaners. Nevertheless, many, if not most, of our patients will fall short of our aims for them. And yet it is important to emphasize here that most of our patients will have a greatly improved gingival condition, some even demonstrating complete resolution of the inflammation. It thus appears obvious that the tissue resistance of most of our patients can cope with a certain amount of residual plaque and this would indicate that the dentist or hygienist should not make a spot judgment on the first visit as to how much training in oral hygiene methods a patient requires. It will be necessary to assess the patient's response over a few visits, and perhaps even after a few months at a recall visit. It will become apparent after a visit or two just how much effort or thoroughness of plaque removal is required for each patient. There are some who will have little gingival inflammation and perhaps no caries, but a notable amount of plaque around the teeth; others will have a minimal amount of adherent micro-organisms and yet may demonstrate acute inflammation. We must therefore modify our approach to each patient depending on the reaction observed.

It must be stressed to the teacher of oral hygiene that terms such as 'correct (or incorrect) brushing' should not be used. There is no right or wrong way to brush the teeth. The result is more important than the method. Therefore, if a patient declares that he can remove plaque and debris using a method of his own, and can show that this method is effective, we would be wrong to insist that he cleans his teeth *our* way. We are therefore concerned with *effective* brushing. Patients often say, 'But my teeth can't be dirty, I brush 20 times a day'. The reply to this remark is, 'It's like having 20 tickets to a lottery. They are all wasted except the one that wins.'

A purely mechanical demonstration of toothbrushing is doomed to failure with most patients. It is necessary to explain to the patient just why he or she is being asked to carry out procedures which are sometimes quite difficult and also time-consuming. The explanation should not just be a general one, but should relate to the patient's problem and be an actual part of the presentation.

Motivation

The nature of plaque and its adhesion to the tooth is carefully explained. The role played in caries and periodontal disease is outlined. At this stage the patient, without having had any toothbrush demonstration, should have been motivated.

Education

The fact that there is not one single 'right' way to brush is emphasized. The right way is any one of a number of different methods which will suit the particular patient.

At this stage the teeth are painted with a disclosing solution and the plaque adhering to the teeth is pointed out to the patient. This indicates the areas which have been missed during home brushing up to now. The plaque is gently scraped off a tooth with the side of a probe to demonstrate how easy it is to remove mechanically.

A suitable brush is selected for the patient and he is told that this is his brush which will be sealed up and kept for training at every visit. Therefore, it is advisable to purchase brushes which are supplied in containers which can be reclosed. (Such a brush, for example, is Oral B 40, or Wisdom Multituft.)

Demonstration

The patient is asked to bring the brush which has up to the present been used at home, but not to buy a new one. It is examined for suitability and the patient is then asked to demonstrate completely how the usual brushing is carried out. It should be emphasized that as complete a brushing as usual is desired. It is of help to set a stop watch at the start. After observing the patient's routine the time to completion is announced (this is usually of the order of 20–30 seconds, although the brusher often insists that he has taken 2 minutes!).

Errors in brushing, areas omitted, lack of organized method are pointed out. An almost constant error is that patients wet the toothbrush before starting. They should be told that this is an

Fig. 17. Division of jaw into 12 brushing areas (lingual and labial). Each area is brushed completely before going on to the next.

Fig. 18. This placement is incorrect. Here the tips of the bristles press against the teeth but cannot adapt to the shape of the teeth and therefore do not enter the embrasures. It matters not whether the patient brushes up and down or across with this placement. There would be the same lack of effect and potential for damage.

incorrect thing to do, and the much worse procedure, the use of hot water, will damage the bristles. Life-size models are used for individual toothbrush demonstration. (Giant size models are not advised unless demonstrating to a large class.)

Each quadrant is divided into three areas, posterior, middle and anterior, and for brushing purposes these are further subdivided into buccal/labial side and lingual or palatal side (*Fig.* 17). The patient is recommended to brush each of these six areas with 8

a

b

Fig. 19. *a*, Correct placement of brush to adapt to shape of teeth and gingivae. *b*, The lower lingual region is often difficult to brush effectively. The 'split bristles' method shown here is useful —the patient may bite down on the back of brush.

strokes of the brush—thus making a total of 48 strokes for each quadrant or approximately 200 strokes for a complete mouth. It has been found that, as noted above, the patient has little concept of time taken for brushing but can readily count 200 strokes.

39

Furthermore, the strokes relate to specific areas of the mouth while, even if say a timer is provided (e.g. egg timer), there is no guarantee that the patient will brush any more methodically.

There are many brushing methods. The dentist or hygienist should not overcomplicate by using too many different techniques, but should be able to demonstrate at least two methods (*Figs.* 18, 19).

a

b

Fig. 20. Bending the handle of a toothbrush in order to assist in cleansing the anterior teeth. However, this unnecessarily overcomplicates the procedure and the patient needs two brushes at least.

The 'Roll' Technique

Effective toothbrushing techniques are not easily acquired by the average patient. Therefore exotic and overcomplicated manoeuvres should be avoided. Perhaps most widely taught (routinely) is the 'roll' method although this still offers difficulties to those who lack manual dexterity, patience or who have limited wrist movement. The brush is placed on the first of our twelve designated sectors of the jaw with the bristles on the alveolar mucosa pointing away from the occlusal surface. The side of the bristles press against the attached gingiva and sulcus area. The bristles are then rolled across the gingiva toward the occlusal keeping the sides of the bristles pressed firmly against the tissues (they should appear to blanch) and with many of the bristles sweeping through the embrasures. This stroke is repeated eight times in each region. Assuming that the buccal area was brushed, this is followed by the lingual and repeated around the whole arch. The occlusal surfaces are then brushed with a to-and-fro action. The emphasis in all the brushing is that the brush should be used as a broom to sweep, not as a scrubbing brush to scour. The brush is often held vertically for the lingual surfaces of the upper and lower incisor teeth. Some dentists bend the handle of the brush to facilitate this action (*see Fig.* 20).

The Bass Technique

This is one of the techniques which has become more popular and is dependent on the use of fine plastic multitufted brushes. The brush is applied in the same section by section pattern as previously but with the bristle direction at an angle of 45° to the long axis of the teeth and pointing toward the gingival sulcus. The bristles in fact are made to enter the sulcus and the brush rotated firmly in a small circle without moving the bristle ends from the crevice. In this way the gingival areas of the tooth and the 'pockets' are cleaned. The action is repeated in adjacent areas following the previously described pattern. Some dentists advocate a to-and-fro motion of the bristles in the sulcus area instead of the circular motion. There would appear to be little to choose between the two actions. The lingual areas of the anterior teeth are brushed using the same action but holding the brush head vertically.

The Charters Technique

This is nowadays not used so often as the Bass method and consists of a substantially similar action except that the brush is placed with the bristles pointing occlusally at an angle of 45°, i.e. there is no action of bristle in the gingival sulcus but the vibrating motion concentrates on cleaning the proximal embrasures.

These various methods should not be taught to the patients indiscriminately but the patient's ability to achieve successful plaque removal with the simplest methods should first be evaluated and

41

here differences in tooth alignment, arch form and size, inclination and manual ability may bring about modification in teaching methods. This emphasises the need for personal 'one-to-one' training and the disadvantages of group 'teach-ins'.

Assessment

After each demonstration the patient is asked to brush his own teeth similarly, and the dentist or hygienist may help by placing the patient's brush in the correct position and helping to guide the wrist or hand action.

Following this disclosing agents are used and the amount of residual plaque is demonstrated.

A similar procedure is adopted on the following visit approximately one week later, with the disclosed plaque indicating areas which have been overlooked.

Further training is given and it is common for sufficient ability and control to take three to four visits to achieve.

Dentifrices

Although the removal of debris and plaque from the tooth surfaces and gingivae is almost entirely a mechanical one, the importance of a good dentifrice should not be minimized. A recent report (Consumer's Association, 1974) on dentifrices by an independent non-dental organization was widely publicized as proclaiming that toothpastes were unnecessary as it was 'the brush that did the cleaning'. The readers were also advised to buy the cheapest toothpaste they could get (preferably fluoride containing) and the bargain offers of the local supermarket were recommended.

As dentists and professional advisers we should be more responsible. Our patients expect a little more advice than 'use the one which has the taste that you prefer' or 'use the cheapest you can get'.

While we need not necessarily choose one particular brand to recommend to our patients, it is sensible to name two or three which we believe to be safe and useful, and which are believed to have a constantly maintained formulation. One of the dangers of recommending 'supermarket toothpastes' is that they are often 'own brand' products made by unknown manufacturers and sometimes sold on a temporary basis while they are profitable or popular. Without the name of a reputable manufacturer, whose existence depends on maintaining a hard-won and expensively earned public acceptance, the product can be dropped or its formula changed to a more profitable one.

The dentifrices which are usually worth recommending purely from a therapeutic standpoint are those which contain fluoride compounds, and have been developed and marketed after careful research and testing.

Special Purpose Dentifrices

Some patients who have sensitive cervical areas on their teeth may benefit from the use of desensitising pastes such as Sensodyne or Emoform (Thermodent). Although many patients state that they have been advised to use these pastes to treat gingivitis or periodontitis, there is no justification for such a recommendation. The only possible value for such dentifrices is in the symptomatic treatment of sensitivity of dentine—not gingivae. Before treating painful areas in this manner a thorough investigation into more definitive causes should be carried out.

When these pastes are used, the patient should be instructed to brush with a small amount on a toothbrush—as they would with a 'normal paste' and then to follow up with a little of the paste rubbed with a finger into the sensitive areas.

OTHER CLEANSING DEVICES

Dental Floss (Fig. 21)

Dental floss may be either waxed or unwaxed. A double width floss, Dentotape is probably easiest for patients to handle, but is still not available in the U.K. There is at present a vogue for unwaxed floss because it is said that in use strands open and trap plaque and debris, and hence clean the interdental spaces better. The waxed floss has been used for generations with satisfactory results but in general few patients persevere with the use of either type. Whereas the average patient accepts the use of a toothbrush as part of the daily routine, flossing is not so naturally accepted and considerable difficulty is experienced in handling it. Even if the technique is apparently mastered, enquiry subsequently among our patients has revealed that too many give up after all too short a period.

Technique of flossing

Careful demonstration is always necessary. Written instructions are useful only after there has been practical training and practice in handling. It has been found easier to cut off a six inch length of floss and tie the ends together to form a loop. This is then held as in the illustration (A) between left thumb and right index finger in order to clean the upper left quadrant. The fingers are reversed for the right quadrant. The loop is held as in (B) for the lower teeth. The floss is held taut between the fingers and is gently worked from the occlusal through the contact point down to the gingival crevice where if possible it is slid along the tooth surface just under the crevice and the two hands are brought as near together as possible, thus wrapping the floss around half the circumference of the tooth. In this position

a

b

c

Fig. 21. Using floss: *a*, Holding a loop in position for the upper teeth of left side. *b*, Finger position of loop for lower teeth. *c*, The floss is wrapped around the tooth.

the floss is gently drawn occlusally while being kept firmly against the tooth surface. The action is repeated and then the surface of the neighbouring tooth across the embrasure is similarly treated. The patient is instructed to clean all the proximal surfaces changing grip as indicated. Where it is not possible to introduce the floss through a contact point (e.g. soldered contacts of bridge pontics or splints) the material is passed under the contact using a floss threader (Nupons, Zon, etc).

The patients usually have even more difficulty handling unwaxed floss and it is very doubtful whether any supposed advantage will outweigh the difficulties encountered, or will bring measurable benefits except to the floss salesmen. Hill, Levi and Glickman (1973) demonstrated that there were no significant differences in reduction of interdental plaque and interdental gingival inflammation produced by toothbrushing, and toothbrushing followed by the use of floss, either waxed or unwaxed. There are many flossing devices on the market but none is recommended because they are no easier to handle then the floss itself (*see* Chapter 5).

Fig. 22. Different makes of wood sticks. The firmest are the Portia (toothpicks) on the extreme right. For this reason they surprisingly need fairly wide embrasures between the teeth, because they do not compress. Probably the most acceptable sticks today are the Sanodents (double ended), shown at left.

Wood Sticks (Fig. 22)

Many patients will fairly readily take to the use of wood sticks (Stimudents, etc.—*see* Appendix). These, together with other interdental cleaners of measurable dimensions, should be recommended only where there is sufficient interdental space not filled by gingival tissue. Care is necessary in teaching the use of wood sticks. They should not be used as toothpicks, which is what the patients will tend to do but the stick should be inserted into the embrasure, pointed end first, with the stick at an angle of 45° to the long axis of the tooth, and the sharp edge of the stick away from the gingiva. The stick is rubbed about 12 times in each space with the tip pointing

45

coronally. A methodical approach should be emphasized, that is, the patient should start from a fixed point in the mouth and work round the mouth back to the same point. In fact there should be some order about using the sticks so that no space is missed out. There may be some difficulty in reaching spaces in the posterior part of the mouth, and other devices or techniques may have to be employed. The Portia type of wood sticks (in fact the original idea of toothpicks) are quite inexpensive and may be sufficient for some patients but because they are made of hard wood and do not compress in use, surprisingly they require a little more space than the more compressible Stimudents type of stick.

Fig. 23. *a,* Small Interspace (embrasure) brush compared with, *b,* conventional toothbrush.

Fig. 24. Method of use of Perio-Pak or Perio-aid with inter-changeable 'bottle wash' type brushes.

Inter-dental Brushes (Figs. 23, 24)

The Halex inter-space brush or the Jordan Inter-brush (*see fig.* 23) have the advantage that they will reach the posterior areas easily and patients do not often have difficulty in their use. They have the advantage of being reasonably inexpensive. It is also possible to clean the embrasures from both lingual and labial aspects of the jaws, other small brushes may be disposable and attached to metal handles by a screw ring (Perio aid, Periopak). They are usually expensive—the bottle-washing type of brush does however remove plaque from the posterior teeth very easily; and a similar brush which can be employed, is the small type of brush which is marketed for cleaning the blades of electric shavers. All are used by entering the embrasures at the same angle as recommended with the wood sticks.

Fig. 25. Gauze strips may be very satisfactory if the spaces are wide enough.

Gauze Strips (Fig. 25)

If the spaces between the teeth are wide, the proximal surfaces of the teeth may be cleaned by half inch gauze strips (ribbon gauze would be ideal).

Polishing Cloths

Polishing cloths may be used (thin towelling cut to the shape of the fingers, and sometimes sewn to an average shape by dental staff in possible unoccupied moments) to polish the surfaces of all teeth before brushing. However, this would seem to be a further complication for the already burdened patient but may be reserved as a special armamentarium for the difficult case, e.g. the handicapped child, and here it may be much easier for the mother or other attendant to use a cloth than a brush.

47

REFERENCES

American Dental Association Council on Dental Materials and Devices (1974). Withdrawal of acceptance of Water Pik oral irrigating device. *J. Am. Dent. Assoc.* **89**, 1178.

Arnim S. S. (1963) The use of disclosing agents for measuring tooth cleanliness. *J. Periodontol.* **34**, 227.

Brasch S. V., Lazarou J., Van Abbe and Forrest J. O. (1969) The assessment of dentifrice abrasivity in vivo. *Br. Dent. J.* **127**, 119.

Consumers' Association (1974) Report on Dentifrices. *Which?* February, p. 36.

Hill H. C., Levi P. A. and Glickman I. (1973) The effects of waxed and unwaxed dental floss on interdental plaque accumulation and interdental gingival health. *J. Periodontol.* **44**, 411–413.

Horowitz H. S. and Lucye H. S. (1966) A clinical study of stannous fluoride in a prophylaxis base and as a solution. *J. Oral Ther.* **3**, 17.

Kanai S. (1966) The effect of burnishing on the margins of occlusal amalgam fillings. *Acta Odontol. Scand.* **24**, 47, 53.

Löe H. and Schiott C. Rindom (1970) The effect of chlorhexidine on the development of dental plaque and gingivitis in man. *J. Periodontol.* **5**, 79.

Massler M. (1969) Teenage cariology. *Dent. Clin. North Am.* **13**, 412.

Messing J. J. and Ray G. R. (1972) *Operative Dental Surgery.* London, Kimpton.

Riethe P. (1974) The quintessence of mouth hygiene. Berlin, Quintessence.

CONTROL OF THE COMMON DENTAL DISEASES

PART 1: PREVENTION OF CARIES

FLUORIDES IN THE PREVENTION OF DENTAL CARIES

IT has been stated earlier that primary prevention, i.e. protecting against the onset of disease, is far superior to the hitherto practised treatment of incipient disease by drilling and filling. The smallness of a filling gives one no assurance that the margins will not undergo microleakage, whatever the material. Someone once described all filling margins as coming within a classification of: (*a*) Poor (*b*) Poorer, (*c*) Poorest!

There are basically four factors involved in the initiation of dental caries:

1. The susceptibility of the tooth surface to acid attack.
2. Plaque attached to the tooth surface.
3. The bacterial activity in the plaque.
4. Carbohydrate ingested into the plaque.

The interaction of these factors is illustrated by the simplified equation:

$$\underset{\text{Bacteria}}{\overset{\text{Plaque}}{}} + \text{Sucrose} = \text{Acid} + \text{Susceptible tooth surface} = \text{Caries}$$

It would appear that elimination of any one of these would diminish or prevent onset of caries. The prevention of plaque formation on the tooth surface would give a considerable measure of control of bacterial population and would also decrease the ability of the sucrose to be maintained in tooth contact. The control of plaque is discussed elsewhere, but it always creates the dilemma that the patient's maximum co-operation is involved, just as it is if carbohydrate limitation is attempted. Increasing the resistance of the tooth surface enamel against acid products remains the most important means at present which can control dental caries without placing too great a demand on the patient. Heifetz and Suomi (1973) state that many of the measures now advocated for the control of dental disease may be suitable for highly motivated patients but they question whether they are applicable to a wide-scale public health programme. They say that merely possessing a correct attitude is not the same as taking the necessary action. The capability to induce mass behaviour change through public health programmes is still not available. When asked how successful we have been in changing the habits of the population in regard to sweets and in-between snacks, we are bound to answer, 'Not at all'. They go on to say that the greatest 'pay-off' in terms of wide-scale control of oral disease exists in capitalizing as heavily as possible on preventive measures which by-pass individual co-operation or keep it at best to a minimum.

FLUORIDATION OF WATER SUPPLIES

The resistance of the enamel surface of the tooth to acid attack can be very greatly enhanced by the incorporation of minute amounts of fluoride ion so that the hydroxyapatite crystals become hydroxy-fluoroapatite.

The formation of this solubility resistant form explains the mode of action of fluorides as preventive agents. The fluoride-enriched enamel may be found in the outer layers to the extent of 30–40 microns, with the highest fluoride levels nearest the surface. This would account for the ability of fluorine compounds to act topically, a process of diffusion and exchange taking place at the surface and this is also taking place between the salivary ions and the enamel surface. Thus, there is a two-way passage through the enamel surface 'membrane' but if the fluoride ions are somehow combined with salivary agents to form non-ion soluble compounds or are otherwise lost with similarly lost Ca ions then the resistance of the tooth surface will be decreased. Similarly an increase in salivary F ions from outside sources will tend to increase the flow of ions inwards and hence increase the hydroxyfluoroapatite content.

In the child, the developing tooth will receive its necessary building materials from the blood plasma and thus the enamel fluorine content will at this point be completely dependent on systemically absorbed fluorine. After tooth eruption maturation of the enamel takes place and there is considerable evidence that a great deal of fluoride uptake is a topical one. Thus it may be assumed that fluoride acts in two complementary ways—by systemic action and by its topical action.

'CARIES SUSCEPTIBILITY TESTS'

The dentist or his staff may use tests such as the Snyder test to illustrate the existing condition of caries susceptibility in the mouth. The test (and there are many modifications of it) uses a colour indicator to show the amount of acid formed by micro-organisms in a carbohydrate medium and thus measures the quantity of micro-organisms which are capable of acting on carbohydrates to convert them to acids. It is doubtful whether the claimed degree of relationship between actual caries activity and the test results can be relied upon, but it has been suggested that anyway the tests may be used as a patient education aid in motivation for sucrose reduction. This writer, however, has some reservations regarding the ethics of using such tests (which may be costly in materials and time) which have a doubtful diagnostic value but are substitute teaching aids. However, those who may be interested may purchase test kits and instructions from some dental supply houses.

To summarize, the dentist's or hygienist's attitude to the possibility of changing any patient's diet should not be too optimistic. If it were universally and immediately possible the problem of dental disease would be solved overnight. However, the dental team should not under-estimate what can be achieved by enthusiasm, constant repetition, careful teaching of young patients—the younger the better—and of course parental example.

The measure which, in view of the foregoing, brings the greatest benefit in terms of caries control from all aspects is fluoridation of public water supplies, i.e. ensuring an optimum level of 1 ppm of fluoride. An enormous amount of careful research has been carried out for three decades or more on the safety, efficacy and cost of this measure and an overwhelming mass of favourable evidence has been published. Those who may be subjected to anxious questions by members of the public who have been bombarded by objectors are referred to a recent review published in reply to an attack on fluoridation in a national newspaper (Burt, 1973).

The long-term effects are greatest if the optimum fluoride level in water is available from birth. Children pass to adulthood with an increased number of sound healthy teeth. The total need for restorative dentistry is reduced, and those fillings which are necessary are usually simple.

The dentist in practice may question his connection with fluoridation of water supplies. He must be aware that this measure would make his own work much easier, and combined with his own preventive attitude will bring a new dimension and change to his practice. What the dentist in the U.K. can do usefully as far as this measure is concerned is to join the Fluoridation Society (for a small annual fee) and in so doing will add support to the strenuous efforts being made to introduce the benefits to more and more of the population. The dentist will also gain by having access to a large quantity of published material for education of the public and also, if he becomes more involved, for the information of his local authorities.

FLUORIDE TABLETS

In the absence of controlled adequate fluoride levels of public water supplies much consideration has been given to the daily supply of fluoride tablets (usually 2·2 mg, giving a fluoride dose of 1·00 mg daily). Investigations have shown substantial reduction in dental caries with deciduous and permanent dentition when consumption of the tablets has been started early enough. However, it has often been shown that even where tablets are provided without charge there is an eventual 'drop out', with only a small percentage of parents persisting with daily dosage to their children.

In view of the benefits derived from these tablets Davies (1973) strongly recommends that when fluoridation of water is impracticable dentists, doctors and child health clinics should be encouraged to prescribe them. He adds that countries with a national health service should consider including fluoride tablets as a pharmaceutical benefit. An alternative procedure would be to arrange for distribution of the tablets through kindergartens and schools.

It must, of course, be borne in mind that when consideration is given to prescribing or distributing tablets it is essential to ascertain the fluoride content of the water supply in the recipient's area of residence. It is not sufficient to base distribution on the known fluoride level of the water in the dentist's area. Dosage should then be adjusted to the known natural fluoride residential level, with of course no tablet prescription when this reaches a level of 1 ppm. The usual dosage is $\frac{1}{2}$ tablet daily (0·5 mg F) in a fluoride free area for children up to 3 years of age and 1 tablet (1·0 mg F) daily for children over 3 years of age.

Mothers should be warned to keep the tablets out of reach of children, to avoid accidental overdosage. For this reason fluoride tablets disguised as sweets are to be deprecated.

TOPICAL FLUORIDES

The dentist newly entering the field of preventive dentistry tends to believe that this part of the text is the real 'meat' of prevention. One hopes that the previous chapters have convinced him that 'putting something on the teeth', whether it be fluorides or fissure sealants, is only a part of the preventive picture. There is abundant literature evaluating the effects of topical fluoride solutions on the teeth. Bernier and Muhler (1966) list 219 references on the effect of various forms of topical fluoride therapy.

The three main fluoride agents are:

1. Sodium fluoride (NaF), usually applied as a 2 per cent solution in distilled water.
2. Stannous fluoride (SnF_2), usually in an 8 or 10 per cent solution.
3. Acidulated phosphate-fluoride solution or gel (1·23 per cent fluoride ion).

1. *Sodium Fluoride*

The first report of a clinical study using NaF was made by Bibby in 1944. He used a 0.1 per cent solution and gave three applications which resulted in a caries reduction of 30 per cent after one year. The use of 2 per cent solution was first reported by Knutson and Armstrong in 1943, and since that time there have been many trials with results giving annual caries reductions of up to 69 per cent DMFS (decayed, missing and filled surfaces).

The sodium fluoride is stable but should preferably be kept in a plastic bottle. The 2 per cent solution can be made up conveniently by the local pharmacist and is obviously a readily available and inexpensive product. This is a great advantage.

Technique

In all topical fluoride techniques it is recommended that the teeth be cleaned prior to fluoride application. A harsh abrasive prophylactic paste should be avoided (*see* p. 28) and it is recommended that one of the proprietary fluoride-containing pastes be used. Dental floss should be passed through the contact points to remove any plaque or debris in the proximal areas.

Following this the teeth are isolated with cotton wool rolls, a quadrant at a time, and a high speed evacuator is placed in position. The cleaned, isolated teeth are dried by further use of the air syringe and the teeth are then constantly wetted with the sodium fluoride for a period of 4 minutes. After each quadrant is completed the patient is allowed to spit and then the other quadrants are completed in turn. At the termination of the total application the patient is allowed to spit and rinse once only. Average application time is 10 minutes.

The routine use of sodium fluoride 2 per cent would appear to have been largely superseded by the other fluorides but there is no doubt that if no other agent had been introduced we should still be able to obtain very considerable reductions of new caries increments.

It must be stressed here that there are many conflicting reports showing superiority of one type of fluoride over another, but no consensus of opinion from the various trials can be obtained. The conclusions which can be made are that all the mainly used fluorides do affect considerable reductions in DMFS. The differences between them may be marginal and as each type has its staunch advocates the use of a particular agent is often a matter of individual choice, based on convenience, comparative cost and availability. This will be discussed later.

2. *Stannous Fluoride*

A solution of 10 or 8 per cent in distilled water is applied to the teeth for 2 minutes.

Considerable work was carried out with stannous fluoride by Muhler and his co-workers in Indiana. Their findings suggested a much enhanced effect in caries reduction over sodium fluoride but this has not always been confirmed by other workers. However, the following are some properties of the stannous fluoride solution.

1. It is very active and therefore loses its potency rapidly and must be freshly mixed, therefore, by the dentist or his assistant for each application session.
2. It is claimed that stannous fluoride is more effective in adults than NaF.
3. It seems to have effects even in those areas where there is optimum water fluoridation.
4. It tends to stain incipient carious lesions and there is objection to the pigmentation produced.
5. There is a metallic taste which some patients find objectionable.
6. Muhler claimed that a single yearly application of 8 per cent stannous fluoride was sufficient to give caries protection.
7. Further studies tend to show that less than the usual 4-minute exposure given with most topical agents will give effective caries reduction. Mercer and Muhler (1964) reported good results with 30-second treatments, while Scola and Ostrom (1968) further reduced the application time to 15 seconds with similar reported success. Shannon (1972) has reported the development of a stable stannous fluoride 0·4 per cent gel (water-free) with glycerin which shows exceptional promise. If this is indeed successful the low stannous fluoride concentration will be much more acceptable from a taste aspect.

Technique for Stannous Fluoride Topical Applications

A stannous fluoride kit can currently still be obtained (in the U.K.) from Messrs Procter & Gamble for a small charge. When this is used in our practice we always make up a 10 per cent solution.

One gram of stannous fluoride crystals is dissolved in 10 ml of distilled water—a reasonably accurate measuring spoon for 1 g is supplied with the kit. A 10 ml discarded hypodermic syringe makes a convenient measure for the water which is then added to the crystals which have been poured into a small bottle and the mixture is shaken until there is a clear solution.

The teeth are cleaned and polished as described previously. A personal preference is for a stannous fluoride zirconium silicate paste (such as Zircate treatment paste). Cotton rolls are applied to isolate a quadrant (or sometimes both quadrants on the same side). The solution is applied to the teeth with a cotton tip, keeping the teeth wet continuously for two minutes. Dental floss is passed through the contact areas to ensure that they are wetted with the solution. Unwaxed floss is usually recommended but it is doubtful whether this really matters. Each quadrant is similarly treated in sequence.

Time taken on average for complete application is 5 minutes.

Comments

This has been the standard topical fluoride technique of my own practice for the past 15 years, but there is no doubt that the acidulated sodium phosphate solutions or gels are being used currently to a far greater extent.

The quoted disadvantages of the stannous fluoride solutions:

1. The pigmentation of some areas of the teeth.
2. The necessity to mix fresh solutions before treatments.
3. Objections to the taste.

1. Pigmentation (brown or black areas) has never been a cause for anxiety. The staining is associated with incipient areas of caries and indicates arrest of the lesion. It is said to be due to the formation of tin phosphate. Areas which were chalky and soft become brown and *hard.* There is some evidence of remineralization. For the beginner in prevention—who may lack confidence in the ability of topical fluoride solutions to protect the teeth—the evidence of the staining of these incipient lesions demonstrates quite dramatically that a positive effect has occurred. *Intact* enamel does not stain.

2. No difficulty has ever been encountered in preparing fresh stannous fluoride solutions. Very little time is taken with ready to hand materials.

3. The objections to taste vary with different patients. Most children do accept the procedure but some make ugly faces. However, there is no reason why the stannous fluoride concentration should not be reduced by half or APF gels may be used for those few who would not tolerate the taste of stannous fluoride. Some advantages of stannous fluoride are the reported high activity of the solution allowing even a 15 or 30 second treatment to be effective. This is important if a child tends to be restless, when a useful application can still be made. Furthermore, because of this it has never been found necessary to use special applicators or trays. The material because of its distribution method is still quite inexpensive.

Acidulated Phosphate Fluoride (APF)
Solution or gel

This is usually a commercially available product containing 1·23 per cent fluoride. It is the most widely available topical fluoride agent and it is probably now the most widely used. A 4-minute treatment is advised for each area treated. The gels often have added flavours, e.g. orange, grape, lime.

Technique (Fig. 26)

This follows the same pattern as previously described. However, it appears that the 4-minute treatment is rigidly recommended and it

Fig. 26. *a*, Applicators for APF gels or solutions. *b*, Contains a foam material and comes in full or half arch sizes.

is often recommended that special applicators be used to hold the gel or solution in place for the required time. In this way either the lower or upper jaw can be completed in one 4-minute period; and with some applicators the whole mouth may be treated at once. *Average application time* 10 *minutes.*

It is difficult to be dogmatic about the superiority of any one of these solutions. The preventive dentist must make his own choice but may well decide for the APF solution or gel mainly because it is readily available from so many dental supply houses and is well advertised.

In view of the fairly marginal differences a cynic might explain that the popularity of the APF materials is due to the fact that the other two solutions are quite unprofitable from a commercial viewpoint. The high cost of APF solutions as sold by the dental supply houses (in effect 98 per cent water) would not seem to be justified.

Davies (1973) states that the best results using combination treatment were obtained by using a three point programme: (1) Stannous fluoride prophylaxis paste, followed by (2) Topical application of stannous fluoride, and to advise (3) Home use of a stannous fluoride dentifrice. He estimates that this is probably the most economic community approach (other than water fluoridation).

One's own view is that this is substantially correct and any practice adopting this routine would obtain excellent results in preventing dental caries. In our own practice we have returned to the use of topical stannous fluoride after 2–3 years with APF gels and solutions.

Notes for Clinical Practice

1. Topical application of fluoride should be carried out 3 times a year because this is usually made to coincide with school vacations. Parents are taught, 'School holidays means dentist'—this is fundamental to our preventive practice. Thus repeat intervals have a meaning as compared to 6-monthly visits which in the U.K. at least are not related to the school timetable. (To relieve congestion we also relate some visits to 'every half term'.)

2. Topical applications must start with the deciduous teeth and preferably at age $2\frac{1}{2}$–3 years. Again this has been found to be fundamental to preventive practice.

3. Only part of the visit is spent in applying topical agents. A similar amount of time should be spent on instruction or training in dental health care and diet.

There would seem to be some agreement that the effectiveness of topical fluoride treatments is of the order of 30–45 per cent caries reduction.

However, most trials have been necessarily carried out on a limited basis, say over two years, and mostly on children at school, i.e. a captive population. The dentist in practice should be able to improve on the above percentage figures by starting his treatments on the pre-school age children as recommended.

Other Methods of Fluoridation

The practising dentist should be aware of alternative methods for a number of reasons.

1. Patients will question him about them and their efficacy and practicability. He should be able to discuss the pros and cons.
2. It may be that the family live in an isolated area with no possibility of water fluoridation or regular visits to the dentist for preventive attention.
3. Alternative methods may be introduced into the patient's community.

Fluoride Mouth Rinses

Despite some initial equivocal reports on the efficiency of fluoride rinses there is available a considerable amount of evidence of their efficiency when carried out on a mass controlled basis. Studies have shown that supervised regular rinsing (every week or fortnight) with 0·2 per cent sodium fluoride, stannous fluoride or APF solution will reduce the amount of dental decay.

The principle to be noted here is frequent rinsing with very dilute solutions. This is almost an inverse ratio. Further research continues and a definite method that is generally applicable requires to be formulated. Bearing in mind that mouth rinsing trials may be in progress at some schools the dentists should make enquiries about other sources of fluoride before he himself either provides or prescribes further fluoridation.

Fluoride in Milk

There is some pressure in this country from a few sources to provide fluoride in milk. Studies have shown some effectiveness but there are a number of counter arguments (such as that the responsibility for protection is thrust back on the parent) and further much more carefully controlled research is required.

Fluoride in Pregnancy

Some expectant mothers enquire whether supplements taken before the birth of the child will help in the development of the infant's teeth. There is some conflict as to whether there is any reasonable passage of fluoride ion across the fetal barrier. In the U.S.A. products that claim to prevent decay in babies still unborn are banned as not proved effective.

FISSURE SEALANTS

Considerable interest has been aroused by the reported use of sealants in fissures, pits and defects in the enamel surfaces of teeth in order to prevent dental plaque accumulation in these vulnerable areas which could lead to a carious lesion. Although much has now been published about these materials, especially of laboratory trials, the clinical results published have been limited by the short duration of the observations. There is, however, some evidence that *if* the material is correctly applied and *if* it effectively seals the fissures without leakage, then a reduction of fissure caries has been observed over the one or two year periods of the trials.

A great number of dentists who have been involved in prevention, especially on a clinical basis, doubt the true efficacy of, or necessity for, these fissure sealants, and their arguments are based, among others, upon the following reasons:

1. Use of fissure sealants does not eliminate the need for the use of topical fluorides.

2. The fissure sealant, even if effective, protects one surface of the tooth mainly (the occlusal). The other four surfaces at risk (the mesial, distal, buccal and lingual) are dependent on the effect of fluorides and of plaque control by the patient.

3. Many observers experienced in the use of topical fluorides over a number of years, especially with the use of stannous fluoride, do not agree with the advocates of fissure sealants who claim that fluorides are ineffective or of little effect in preventing fissure caries.

4. Fissure sealants should be applied only to those fissures which are so deep that they are potentially carious but not in fact affected by caries. There is some argument as to whether 'sealing in' caries would be harmful—if the seal were 100 per cent effective this would probably be safe, but in practice one cannot be sure of 100 per cent sealing. The choice of which fissures to seal may involve a considerable exercise of judgement and some forecasting—or even guesswork—at the expense of the patient.

5. Fissure sealants, therefore, must be regarded as applicable where used only for primary caries prevention, whereas topical fluorides, especially of the stannous fluoride type, may be effective in controlling already initiated caries and in the reversal of small lesions.

6. The application of the sealant material is far from simple and the many papers giving examples of loss rates of some sealants exemplify this.

However, the main factor must be that it is costly in time and procedure to use these materials in relation to the benefit obtained, and in the present controversial situation it may not appear justifiable to some to involve patients in the necessarily high fees entailed. There may be commercial pressure to use these materials because they are expensive and therefore more profitable to sell than topical fluorides.

Types of Sealants

At present there are available a number of different commercial sealants. The majority are based on the BIS–GMA resin (which is also the main ingredient of most of the new composite filling materials). There are differences in the way in which the sealants are polymerized or cured (after being placed in position). The material which clinical evidence has to date shown to have better adhesive and sealing qualities is one which does not harden until it is irradiated by ultra violet light focused on it from a special lamp. It then polymerizes quickly. The other material hardens by a chemical reaction between the mixed components of the applied paste. There would appear to be some doubt currently regarding the safety of the unmodified ultra violet lamp.

Adhesion for all these materials is obtained by partly decalcifying the immediately surrounding enamel surface, usually by the use of 50 per cent phosphoric acid. The acid etches the surface of the enamel dissolving some of the mineral constituents to a depth of 7–10 microns, and this roughens the surface enabling the fluid sealant to flow into the irregularities and on setting there should be a strong bond formed.

If the decision is made to use fissure sealants, the dentist should study very carefully the instructions for use which are issued by the manufacturer of the particular sealant chosen. This advice regarding method of application is likely to be more accurate than any detailed instruction given in this chapter as all the different materials have variations in composition, however slight.

In connection with the current controversy regarding fissure sealants the Editorial comment of the *Journal of Dentistry* (1974) is of interest:

Increased interest in preventive dentistry will no doubt encourage more widespread use of sealants. Some dentists will, on reading the results of research papers, assess the claim of the sealants' effectiveness. These people will also be conscious of the need to choose carefully the cases for treatment, to have a meticulous clinical technique, and to be critical of the postoperative results. Unfortunately, there will be some who will be too easily swayed by advertising. Sad to say, there may also be those who will recommend the technique because of the financial advantages that may accrue from it, since this service is not yet provided under the terms of the National Health Service . . .

Can the meticulous clinical techniques required for the best results be undertaken by dental auxiliaries? If not, can the cost be justified as a public health measure? . . .

The profession should remember that the introduction of sealants was a breach of etiquette since the concept and treatment were advertised directly to the public by the manufacturers and not through the dental profession. It is ethically questionable to advocate a product when its effectiveness remains unproved. Many dentists are eager to jump on the preventive dentistry bandwagon, but who stands to benefit most from fissure sealants: the patient, the dentist, or the manufacturer?

SUMMARY

Primary Prevention of Caries

It must be repeated that effective plaque reduction is a dominant factor in primary caries prevention. The most commonly practised method (see other chapters) and the most generally effective is by the trained use of the toothbrush.

Plaque elimination must be a part of prevention in all stages, primary, secondary and tertiary.

It should be borne in mind that it will be difficult to teach the very young child to brush effectively, and before the onset of disease it is beyond the capabilities or desire of the very young child or adolescent to carry out tedious brushing (or flossing) procedures in the expectation of avoiding some disease in the remote future. Thus motivation must be strong and must be combined with the message and training repeated frequently—at all recall visits. However, fluoridation in all its forms is the prime caries preventive agent, taking precedence even over plaque control in the young child.

Secondary Prevention of Caries

With already established caries, whether newly formed and just detectable or gross, perhaps rampant, caries, attention should be paid first of all to the prevention of new cavities forming. The carious tooth should not be finally filled (the cavities can be dressed) until the 'infection' of dental caries is controlled or eliminated. Analogy: it is useless to fill up the holes in the skirting boards without getting rid of the mice. They will just make new holes!

One of the more important aspects of secondary prevention, detecting the early carious lesion, is careful inspection and this often involves the use of X-rays (in the form of bite-wings) on a routine basis.

REFERENCES

Fluorides

Bernier J. L. and Muhler J. C. (1966) *Improving Dental Practice through Preventive Measures.* St. Louis, Mosby, p. 124.

Bibby, B. G. (1944) Use of fluorine in the prevention of dental caries, II. *J. Am. Dent. Assoc.* **31**, 317.

Burt B. A. (1973) Water fluoridation. *Br. Dent. J.* **135**, 543.

Davies G. N. (1973) Fluoride in the prevention of dental caries—A tentative cost-benefit analysis. *Br. Dent. J.* **135**, 336.

Heifetz S. J. and Suomi J. D. (1973) The control of dental caries and periodontal disease: a fundamental approach. *J. Public Health Dent.* **33**, 2.

Knutson J. W. and Armstrong W. D. (1943) Effect of topically applied sodium fluoride on dental caries experience. *Public Health Rep.* **58**, 1701.

Mercer V. H. and Muhler J. C. (1964) The effect of a 30-second topical stannous fluoride treatment on clinical caries reduction in children. *J. Oral. Ther. Pharm.* **1**, 141.

Scola F. P. and Ostrom C. A. (1968) Clinical evaluation of stannous fluoride in naval personnel. *J. Am. Dent. Assoc.* **77**, 594–597.

Shannon I. L. (1972) Dialogue on preventive dentistry. Chicago, March, p. 156.

Fissure Sealants

Buonacore M. (1970) Adhesives for pit and fissure caries control. *Dent. Clin. N. Am.* **16**, 693.

Eames W. B. (1972) Pit and fissure sealants. *J. Ga Dent. Assoc.* **46**, 20.

Editorial Comment (1974) *J. Dent.* **2**, 91.

McLean J. W. and Wilson A. D. (1974) Fissure sealing and filling with an adhesive glass ionomer cement. *Br. Dent. J.* **136**, 269.

Parkhouse R. C. and Winter G. B. (1971) The fissure sealant containing methyl and cyanoacrylate as a caries preventive agent. *Br. Dent. J.* **130**, 16.

Rock W. P. (1972) Fissure sealants: results obtained with 2 different sealants after 1 year. *Br. Dent. J.* **133**, 146.

Williams B., Casson M. H. and Winter G. B. (1974) A clinical study using a new ultra violet light polymerised fissure sealant. *J. Dent.* **2**, 101.

CONTROL OF THE COMMON DENTAL DISEASES

PART 2: PERIODONTAL DISEASE

DIET AND DENTAL DISEASE

IF it were possible to initiate a perfect and rigid individual plaque control then the vast majority of our patients would never have gingivitis or, later, periodontal disease. This is a dream and the discipline involved may be carefully observed by some but becomes too tedious and lacking in urgency for most adolescent patients. There is the eternal problem of giving regular consideration to something that may occur in years ahead. How many people at 18 years of age voluntarily think about saving for a retirement pension maturing at 60?

We must accept that very few, if any, patients can ever achieve perfect plaque control. We may demonstrate by cleaning the patient's teeth under the ideal conditions with a good light such as we have in the dentist's office, with brushes, cups, various polishing pastes, strips, tape, etc. Now a disclosing solution is applied. Can we ever swear that there will be no tell-tale red stain somewhere? How can a patient do better under home conditions even if fanatical? Therefore we must accept a varying level of plaque control from each patient.

What level of plaque control is acceptable will depend on our enthusiasm, teaching ability, the patient's skill and interest and the tissue susceptibility. This is the key to the periodontal story.

The prevention of plaque accumulation or its regular removal is, in spite of the foregoing, our best method of avoiding periodontal disease, and therefore the most important preventive measure is the effective use of the toothbrush. To date only the mechanical action of the brush has been regularly shown to remove the bacterial and other deposits. Once gingivitis does occur it becomes easier to motivate the patient because then the ill effects of bacterial accumulation on the teeth can be demonstrated. The use of disclosing solutions shows up the plaque, and the associated areas of inflamed gum can then be pointed out. Thus the patient will have a reason for wanting to brush effectively if the relationship between the plaque and the inflammation is understood. It is a matter for regret that our efforts before the onset of disease are not so successful.

In the present concentration on plaque and plaque control the role of careful scaling is regrettably being minimized. Calculus, whether it is supragingival or subgingival, is the supreme plaque retainer. If calculus is not removed the success of any brushing instruction is prejudiced. It is also unfair to expect the patient to carry out home care procedures which are always quite difficult for some if the teeth are left in a roughened state either through lack of polishing or because calculus still remains. This is not to say that we should not begin brushing instruction from the first oral hygiene visit. But we should also at the same time help the patient in our way by beginning to clean and polish the surfaces of all teeth. Thus careful scaling is a most important factor in the prevention of periodontal disease. It is also a factor in the maintenance of the treated case. No matter how well we teach our patients to carry out plaque elimination procedures most will still form calculus in some regions and will require regular thorough scaling.

Attention must be paid to other causes of plaque accumulation. These are factors which should be dealt with by the dentist when possible; otherwise special methods may be required to be taught to the patient. Some of these causes (e.g. filling overhangs) are listed in Chapter 3 (p. 25).

Many of these conditions are discovered only by careful examination. The regular sensible use of X-rays is important and it is again emphasized here that the newer methods of panoramic mouth surveys are becoming increasingly important.

PERIODONTAL DISEASE

The approach to periodontal treatment may be outlined as follows:

1. Awareness by the dentist and the periodontist of the problem.
2. Informing the patient.
3. Awareness by the patient of the nature of the problem and the patient's reaction to this awareness.
4. Full diagnostic procedure, including detailed past and present medical and dental history. Diet and habit check;
5. Preliminary treatment planning discussion with the patient. Initial patient personality evaluation at this point.
   Assessment of degree of comprehension, i.e. patient's dental I.Q. and manual ability (e.g. arthritic?).
6. Initial therapy:
   Education, motivation and training in home-care methods, plus dentist's or hygienist's treatment of local factors.
7. Reassessment:
   Allocation:
   Patient co-operation good:
   a. No further active treatment necessary
   or
   b. Definitive completion treatment may now begin.

Patient co-operation poor:
Proceed no further, but may refer back for further training if thought desirable.

We should consider these points in detail:

1. *Awareness by the Dentist of the Periodontal Problem*

It is not the purpose here to go into this fully, but it has been frequently demonstrated that one of the main factors in tooth loss is the non-recognition of established periodontal disease by the regularly attended dentist. To be able to treat periodontal disease we must recognize its presence and preferably recognize it early.

2. *Informing the Patient*

It follows that the patient must be informed of the presence of disease and must be fully acquainted with the importance of dealing with it. If this is ignored the patient's fundamental role will be neglected. All too often patients present with advanced disease stating that years ago, when they complained of bleeding gums, they were told that they have 'a little gum trouble' and to—

- *a.* Use an oxygen liberating mouthwash (e.g. Bocasan, Amosan) daily, or
- *b.* Use an intermittent water pressure irrigation device (e.g. Water Pik), or
- *c.* 'You have pyorrhea—nothing can be done. It's just a matter of hanging on until they have to be extracted. In the meantime, we will continue with your fillings.'

In spite of this the disease progresses. The patient has had no information of value because the dentist had none to give. Sometimes, however, the dentist has been well aware of the extent of the problem but has been too embarrassed to tell the patient that, in spite of regular 6-monthly check-ups for ten years, there now appears to be a state of advanced periodontal breakdown. It requires courage, but the extent of the problem should be explained quite clearly to the patient. *We must be careful in our communication with the patient to talk the same language.*

3. *Awareness by the Patient*

Once the patient is aware of the seriousness and extent of the problem there will be some early response, indicating whether there is a strong desire or otherwise to retain the remaining teeth. Often the awareness has been hardened by some periodontal crisis, loss of a loose tooth, or recurrent periodontal abscesses.

4. & 5. *Full Diagnostic Procedures and Preliminary Planning Discussion*

It is beyond the scope of this work to deal with all the diagnostic procedures to be adopted. We are concerned here with those which may modify the treatment plans and the patient's ability to carry them out. It is important to assess the patient's attitude to dental treatment; is there a strong desire to retain the dentition, or would the work involved be a waste of time because the patient really wants complete dentures? A past dental history may reveal other attempts at periodontal treatment, gingivectomies and other surgical procedures. It should be of interest to hear the patient's account as to why they failed. Is the patient competent or willing to carry out home care procedures?

What should be noted are:

a. Untidy, unkempt females, with dirty finger nails, etc. are unlikely to be willing to spend much time on the less visible teeth, unless very strongly motivated.

b. Smoking is a factor in gingival disease and heavy smoking, especially in the young, will prejudice or delay a successful outcome to periodontal therapy.

c. Alcoholics often make impossible subjects.

d. There may be a lack of the manual ability necessary to carry out the essential home care, e.g. the patient may be arthritic or otherwise handicapped. There may be a gag reflex, making the usual brushing procedure impossible.

e. Some patients on heavy drug therapy, for example phenytoin, may have difficulties in maintaining concentration except for very short periods.

f. With regard to diet, it has been demonstrated on a number of occasions that the nature of the diet has little effect as a cleansing agent and plaque remover. However, a high sucrose diet is plaque encouraging and the patient should be advised possibly to decrease the high consumption of sucrose. Some dentists may wish to carry out Snyder tests or modifications to reinforce this advice (*see* Section on Diet, p. 76).

g. *Habits.* These may include fingernail, pipe stem and thread biting, mouth breathing and tongue thrusting.

h. *Parafunction.* Bruxism, clenching and 'lazy' mastication, or lack of masticatory ability (open bite) may all require correction. (*Fig.* 27).

Fig. 27. An occlusal bite (or night) guard may be fitted where there is bruxism, or other grinding or clenching habits.

i. Finally, and probably most important, attention should be paid to the patient's emotional state in that it may be the basis for much of the foregoing. It is also clear that many oral manifestations are totally or partially the result of emotional stress. Many workers for example have shown a close relationship between this and acute ulcerative gingivitis. And there is no doubt that conditions such as bruxism, clenching and biting habit often have an origin in stress situations and depression.

6. *Initial Therapy*

At this stage there may be referral to other members of the dental team specially trained to deal with these problems. A dental assistant trained as health educator may initiate the motivation and teaching plan of the programme. Audio-visual aids may be used, but these have very little or no effect unless they are used intelligently, with nearly always a one-to-one relationship with the teacher. Merely sending the patient into an audio-visual room with instruction to: 'watch this' is almost useless, as is filling the waiting room with a mass of pamphlets, booklets, exhortations to do this and that procedure. The teaching of mouth care is a personal one and each patient requires individual attention with a modified approach depending on all the personal idiosyncracies outlined above.

The early stage of dental health care training is often fraught with difficulties. If the dentist is not to carry this out himself, it is important that he does not just dismiss the patient with remarks such as, 'Miss Brown is now going to show you how to clean your teeth'. The response to this from a 60-year-old may well be, 'I am not going to be shown how to brush my teeth at my age by a chit of a girl. Why, I've taught three generations how to brush.' It is the dentist's own responsibility before handing over the patient to assess the patient's brushing ability—one way is to use a disclosing agent and demonstrate the plaque in a mirror held by the patient, emphasizing that however well the patient brushed it was impossible to deal with this invisible coating of bacteria until now, and that specific techniques will be demonstrated. It should then be emphasized that the hygienist or other auxiliary has had very special training in dealing with these problems.

The patient is asked to bring the regularly used toothbrush for the first session with the hygienist or dentist for oral hygiene training. (It should be noted that the term oral hygiene *instruction* is not used.

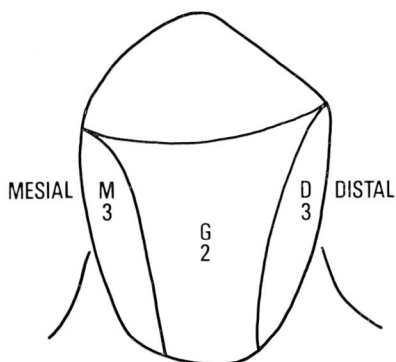

Fig. 28. Diagrams showing methods of scoring in making out a plaque index. Higher scores are given to areas where plaque is nearest to the gingival crevice and would therefore be more harmful.

The patient needs to be *trained* rather than just instructed.) It is pointed out that a new toothbrush should not be bought for this visit. We would like to see the old one in action. At this stage, the patient is asked to brush as if at home, leaving nothing out and taking just as much time as usual. It is useful here to set a stop-watch or timer unobtrusively and then to show the patient the brushing time. For most new and uninstructed patients the average time has been found to be around 25 seconds. After the brushing has been completed, a disclosing solution is applied and the neglected areas are pointed out.

A plaque index may be prepared and done routinely as teaching progresses (*Fig.* 28).

It is tempting at this stage to go straight on to the demonstration of brushing technique. It is important, however, to avoid giving the impression that we are ordering the patient to carry out a number of techniques without understanding. For this reason, some time is spent on describing the nature and the ill-effects of plaque and how it acts on the gum tissue and causes disease. Some colour slides may be used to demonstrate the beneficial effects of plaque removal carried out by other patients. Thus, brushing *technique* in our training

a

b

Fig. 29. Shortening or straightening incisors may take a few moments with a disc. The patient feels happier to brush her more pleasing teeth.

programme assumes a role secondary to motivation and education of the patient. If the patient understands, he or she will want to carry out these procedures. Then it matters not what method is used, as long as the plaque is removed and the patient desires to remove it. We use the code M.E.D.A.R. for our training. This indicates *Motivation, Education, Demonstration, Assessment* and *Re-training*.

Demonstration may be carried out initially on life-size models, but always ultimately the patient must be taught to use the brush effectively in his or her mouth, with suitable corrections by the hygienist or other teacher. There must never be any harsh criticism

a

b

Fig. 30. This patient's home care efforts improved enormously following completion of his restorative work. Note the gingival condition, before and after.

such as 'You are very neglectful' or 'You are careless', but always encouragement.

Many patients often feel that their teeth are in a hopeless condition and that it is just a matter of time before they are lost, so why bother? This is especially the case if the anterior teeth are unsightly or the gums bleed excessively. A tremendous change in patient co-operation can occur after some reshaping of the incisors, replacing an unsightly anterior filling, or a couple of visits spent on removing gross calculus. The dramatic change may convince the patient that treatment is worth while. This again is part of motivation. (*Figs. 29 and* 30.)

It is essential for the dentist to do all he can to make the patient's task easier.

It may well be entirely erroneous to persist with that timeworn injunction to brush after every meal. This encourages the patient to believe that the object of cleaning is food removal and leads both dentist and patient to ignore the dangers of plaque. Effective total

a

b

Fig. 31. This patient was taking high doses of Epanutin (Dilantin, phenytoin). It took one year of persevering toothbrush training (she could not use floss or other materials) to achieve the excellent result without surgery.

71

plaque removal, which should be our goal, if carried out once per day is far better than two or three or even a dozen incomplete manipulations.

Kegeles (1963) has postulated that a four-point scheme should be adhered to where the patient is resistant to training and motivation or is having some difficulty. The patient should come to believe the following statements:

 a. That he is susceptible to periodontal disease.
 b. That periodontal disease is personally serious.
 c. Periodontal therapy and plaque control are beneficial preventive steps to treat or correct the condition.
 d. That the condition occurred due to natural causes and not as a punishment meted out by God for his past sins.

We may then go on to a demonstration of an effective toothbrushing method (not a *correct* method, but an *effective* method) and may be individually tailored to the patient's capabilities. There is no single method of toothbrushing adequate for all cases. Methods are described in another chapter. (*See also Fig.* 31.)

7. *Reassessment*

Perhaps 5 or 6 visits close together may be devoted to motivation and oral hygiene training. During, and at the termination of this phase it will become apparent that the patient is co-operating fully or not at all, with some in-between cases. If there has been full co-operation, the early stages of periodontal disease may have resolved and frequently, at the end of this phase, no further treatment except maintenance will be required.

There may be some patients who although co-operative, do not seem to be progressing satisfactorily or sufficiently rapidly and it becomes apparent that however assiduously they may brush, they do not eliminate sufficient plaque to resolve their gingival inflammation. These patients will require extra attention and possibly accessory aids in their home care. If there is sufficient loss of papillary height for the introduction of wood sticks of the Stimudents Interdens or Sanodents type, the use of these should be taught. They are almost always essential following the surgical phase of periodontal therapy, and patients will usually learn to use them quite readily. (*See* Chapter 3 for details of method.) The use of dental floss may be advised for others with difficult plaque removal problems where sticks are not advisable. Patients do not readily take to the floss habit and many give up after a time, however conscientiously they may have been trained in its use. The various flossing gadgets now being offered seem at first sight to be helpful but they have many disadvantages, principally that they tend to get foul during use. Adjustment of the floss in the holders is difficult and results in tangles and waste. It is often said that the patient who learns to handle these flossing gadgets must perforce have sufficient ability to use floss around the mouth without them!

Otherwise the use of interdental brushes or stimulators may be tried. Such instruments are the Perio-Pak (Crescent) the Halex Interspace brush, the Jordan Inter brush etc. Patients vary in their likes and dislikes of these and on the whole the Interspace brush or the Inter brush are the most acceptable.

Exceptionally, there will be some failures and serious consideration must be given to the termination of treatment at this point—some may be referred back for reconsideration of their problem and further motivation.

The few remaining patients who are completely unco-operative should be informed of the difficulties, and it is often best to set out the reasons tactfully in writing. A letter along the following lines is suggested:

Dear . . .

I am sure that you are aware that we have been very concerned about your dental condition and we have discussed the way in which your mouth can be restored to a healthy state. It has been emphasized that a great deal can be accomplished by your own efforts in daily attention to your mouth and gums using the methods which have been taught here. This is essential if your planned treatment is not to produce a poor result very soon after completion, and in that case you will probably be worse off than if the work had not been carried out.

We often have to spend 5 or 6 visits with a patient before the correct methods can be carried out at home and, as you know, we have been demonstrating this to you.

I am worried about the fact that for some reason you do not seem able to achieve as much success with our methods as we would both like. Obviously you would like to get on with the rest of the dental treatment as keenly as I would be to recommend it.

I therefore feel that we ought to have a discussion as to whether we can plan any changes in our approach, as you would not want to go to the trouble and expense of having dental work done which is doomed to eventual failure.

Yours sincerely

Maintenance

This is a most important but frequently overlooked, part of perio-dontal therapy. It should have been impressed on the patient that there is a susceptibility to periodontal disease. Therefore, at the termination of definitive treatment, by which time the patient should be able to carry out all necessary home care procedures, an appointment for reappraisal should be made at an interval of 1 month. If there is good maintenance the appointment period may become 3 months, then 4 months, but unless the patient has developed an extremely good plaque control method the interval between maintenance recalls should rarely exceed this. A complete retraining is almost always necessary after a year or so.

We must all of us endeavour to lighten the patient's work load in controlling periodontal disease. It should be on the conscience of the profession that we have not yet discovered a means of treating periodontal disease which leaves the patient free to go about his daily living and forget all about us. This should be our aim. We should also not burden him with a mass of oral hygiene appliances, but prescribe the minimum necessary to ensure the simple maintenance of good oral health. It is salutary at this point to remember the report of the Editor of the *New Mexico Dental Journal* in which he says, '1972 has been the year of the great "control programme" boom, and reports are that gingivitis is down but suicides are up, presumably from frustrated flossers choosing the easy way out. We have promised salvation to the faithful, but have struck terror in the hearts of the arthritic and handicapped who cannot possibly pass the stain test.'!

To Summarize

Prevention of periodontal disease involves the following:

1. Plaque prevention or elimination mainly and generally by brushing.
2. Careful inspection at regular intervals for the development of incipient gingival disease—probe gently for pockets.
3. Regular radiographic examination (*Fig.* 32).
4. Regular scaling and careful polishing. Most thorough scalings take more than one visit to complete. The number of visits is determined by the amount and toughness of the calculus and coincidentally by the time taken for instruction and reinstruction of the patient's home care methods.
5. All our patients (almost without exception) will require retraining in brushing and other home care procedures after a year or two. Therefore we must check the patients' technique 'not by asking but by watching' at the regular check-up visits.
6. There should be a regular but simple recall system for all patients who have been and are under periodontal care.
7. Consideration of gingival health when carrying out restorative procedures (crowns, inlays, etc.). The crown margins should be supragingival where possible.

a

b

Fig. 32. The importance of regular radiographic investigation is emphasized here. The gingiva at casual examination appear to be healthy—pink, stippled, knife edge margins. The suspicious sign is the drifting lateral incisor. *b*, Radiographs reveal a diastrous situation.

Conclusion

We can nearly always control gingivitis so as to prevent its progression to *periodontitis* and attain a return to a healthy gingival state. Our problem is that this requires constant vigilance and hard work from the patient and the dental team. Very few preventive measures will succeed on a community basis if we place the responsibility on the individual member of the public. Therefore what we must hope for is a periodontal equivalent of fluoride (especially water fluoridation) which reduces dental decay incidence without patient responsibility.

75

DIET AND DENTAL DISEASE

The difference between nutrition and diet should be appreciated. We may say that on the whole the population of this country do not suffer from nutritional disorders in the way that many of the populations do of the underdeveloped countries.

For correct nutritional needs there should be a balanced intake of foods such as meat, fruit, vegetables, milk and bread. These in reasonable rations will provide the protein, fat and carbohydrates plus the minerals and vitamins necessary for health. In describing someone as suffering from malnutrition it is not necessarily implied, although this is often inferred, that there is insufficient intake of food but that the nutritional process is awry, either by excessive or unbalanced intake.

If, however, there is concern regarding the patient's nutritional state, e.g. scurvy, then reference should be made to the patient's physician.

However, the dentist and his team should be concerned with the dietary balance and in particular with advice regarding carbohydrate intake. Plaque formation and hence caries and periodontal disease is considerably increased with high sucrose intakes. The patient should therefore be instructed on the bacterial origins of plaque and on how sucrose takes part in this formation in a number of ways, one of which is by providing nutrition for the bacteria.

The following advice which is probably of use only if often repeated—with explanations of the reasons behind the advice, should be offered:

1. Carbohydrate intake is usually excessive and should be reduced where possible. This will benefit teeth, prevent obesity and perhaps may even delay atherosclerosis.

2. For caries prevention it has been shown that sugar intake restricted to mealtimes will produce a lower caries rate than if sugar is allowed in the form of in-between snacks.

3. Thus emphasis should be placed on the perils of frequency of intake over the 24-hour period being worse (other than from a systemic viewpoint) than the quantity of carbohydrate intake.

4. Substitution of savoury or fruity non-sugary snacks should be tried, especially with children, where it may be possible to avoid cultivation of a 'sweet tooth'. This occurred without doubt during and immediately following the second World War when sweet rationing was present in the U.K. and many children grew up without the daily obsessive desire for candy bars.

5. The type of sugar containing food which is consumed is important. Liquids would appear to be less harmful than sticky

substances which adhere to the tooth surface and there is some evidence that chocolate may be less harmful than, say, toffee. To advise one over the other would appear to interfere with the total philosophy of prevention which is that sucrose is harmful and therefore to discuss marginal differences may not be a rational approach.

REFERENCES

Glickman I. (1972) *Clinical Periodontology*. Philadelphia, Saunders, pp. 443–474.

Goldman H. M. and Cohen D. W. (1973) *Periodontal Therapy*, 5th ed. London, Kimpton, pp. 427–461.

Grant, D. A., Stern I. Q. and Everett F. G. (1972) *Orban's Periodontics*, 4th ed. London, Kimpton, pp. 363–410.

Kegeles S. S. (1963) Some motives for seeking preventive dental care. *J. Am. Dent. Assoc.* **67,** 92.

CHAPTER 6

THE CHILD PATIENT

GENERAL APPROACH

THE relationship between dental practice and the child should be a happy one from the start. The earlier in the child's life that this relationship begins the easier it is to achieve. Thus ideally we should concentrate our efforts on instructing parents on the importance of bringing the pre-school child to the practice. The usual starting age for visits is 2½–3 years. The advantages are many.

1. Very few children at this age will have been exposed to anxiety arising from tales of dental 'horrors'. It would be pleasant to believe that the public image of the dentist as a bloodthirsty sadist with forceps in hand and knee in chest tugging at a howling patient no

Fig. 33. A typical young adult who has had topical fluoride since the age of 2 years. He is one of a host of 20–30-year-olds in our practice who have never known what a dental burr feels like.

longer exists, but regrettably almost all newspaper articles and other mass media publications tend to concentrate on key emotive words such as 'toothache', 'drill', 'blood', 'extractions'. The child who becomes a friend of the practice before coming under this harmful influence will later on reject these accounts of trauma as alien to itself and the practice. Indeed it becomes possible when the child is older to emphasize that the involvement in the preventive approach is one factor which avoids the discomforts which may have then been recounted to him by schoolmates.

2. It is more usual to find at, say, 3 years that any caries attack is minimal or non-existent (although there may be some startling exceptions) and hence very few children will have at this age associated their own teeth with pain. The dentist may therefore go on from this point maintaining a 'non-discomfort' approach for many years.

3. Attendance from pre-school age enhances the value of preventive techniques. There has been no time to acquire bad habits. Indoctrination can be slow and subtle and the child 'grows up with it'. The teeth are all fairly recently erupted into the oral cavity and the uptake of fluoride is enhanced. (*Fig.* 33.)

Some of the dental practitioners' attitudes which often still exist in relation to treatment of children should be discarded or modified. Many dentists still believe that:

1. Parents should be excluded from the 'treatment' room from the start, or as soon as possible, and that the dentist/child relationship is enhanced because of this and the dentist may then himself resolve the problem of cutting the necessary cavities in the teeth.
2. Gifts should not be given to children at the termination of the appointment. It has been said that this is a form of bribery and is therefore wrong.
3. Fillings should be done as soon as they are detected (as pinpoint fillings) because it is relatively painless to drill the cavity form and it 'gets the child used to the drill'.

It is probable that these prohibitions existed because of the unpleasantness of repair dentistry and in order to enable the dentist to carry out his tasks in a calmer atmosphere. The change in attitude to a preventive one almost certainly means a reversal of these views:

1. It is necessary for a parent or responsible adult to be present with the pre-school child at the time of examination and possibly for some visits afterwards. We consider the parents (and we tell them so) to be members of the preventive team and therefore it is necessary to discuss with them the whole field of prevention in relation to their child. Thus at 3 years of age it is rarely possible for a child to grasp the techniques of brushing or the importance of plaque control; neither can eating habits or the merits of food preparations be explained to anyone but a responsible adult. Other aspects of the child such as general health and physical or psychological problems would need to be known and recorded. A regular discussion regarding the child's progress is necessary.

2. Gifts are always given to our young patients unless something is done to affect our 'friendship' on a particular visit. The accusation of bribery does not apply because at no time is a child promised 'sit

still and let me drill the tooth and you will get a present' because rarely is a tooth drilled. A gift is not 'earned' by submitting to trauma but is an expression of a happy relationship such as exists in one's family where gifts are given to sons and daughters because they are loved ones. An indication of this happy relationship is demonstrated by the frequency with which the children bring gifts for the dentist!

3. The presents for the youngest age group are nearly always useful in the sense that they are usually a balloon with a suitable inscribed dental message such as, 'Tommy Tooth says, "Take care of me, I'm hard to replace." '

THE FIRST VISIT

The young child is almost always welcomed by the hygienist who will seat the patient in the chair before the dentist enters and will demonstrate, often with a picture book, some aspect of the teeth. It might even be a children's story with reference to teeth. The dentist comes in at the point where the child is happily seated and may have had some sort of oral examination from the hygienist. A more detailed examination is carried out but very often without the use of a probe. A blunt plastic instrument may be used as some form of a seeker. For the few very apprehensive children the dentist may remove his usual surgeon's coat and approach the child in his 'ordinary clothes'. This gives him a more 'fatherly' appearance, but the occasions when this is necessary are rare. Even rarer are the occasions when the child will need to be examined seated on the lap of a parent in the dental chair, or even away from the dental chair at some more familiar easy chair.

A careful examination should be carried out as soon as it is practicable (it may not be at the first visit) and having due regard to the age of the child, the jaw relationship and development stages should be considered. It is important to look at the teeth in their closed 'centric' position. This is too easily forgotten in the occasional difficult situation of getting the child to 'open'! An O.P.G. (or panoramic X-ray scan) is a very valuable diagnostic aid especially in the child patient, where very full information relating to the complete dentition, both erupted and non-erupted, can be obtained with the advantage that no films are placed in the child's mouth and the radiation dose is considerably reduced compared to conventional intra-oral methods.

It is always better to do some preventive treatment for the child, and most of them will accept a prophylaxis and topical fluoride from the first visit. It may be necessary with a minority to use only a rubber cup revolving slowly over the teeth (after demonstrating its effect on a finger nail).

RECALL VISITS

The parent of a child at school is asked to bring the child for attention at every long school vacation, i.e. at the Christmas, Easter and Summer vacations. This provides an interval of approximately 4 months between visits, giving 3 visits in a year. If, indeed, the parent is impressed with the responsibility of ensuring these regular visits, no recall programme will be required. Recall will, however, be necessary for pre-school children and those who are unable for some reason to attend in the normal vacation times or whose parents are unable to assume this responsibility. Ideally the mother who has been attending the practice as a patient herself will have received instructions regarding the dental health of her child from birth. There will be assessment of fluoride content of the local water supply—this information is readily obtainable from the water company concerned. Regrettably most supplies will be short of the optimum natural level of around 1 ppm and therefore some discussion usually takes place with the parent regarding provision by the mother of some separate fluoride intake for the child in order to make up for this deficiency. There are today a number of methods of achieving this: dissolving F tabs in the child's drinking water, ingestion of tablets, fluoride and vitamin lozenges, etc., and in some countries fluoridated milk or salt. However, by and large most parents do not succeed in maintaining a satisfactory routine because it becomes demanding.

Instructions are given at a later date, i.e. as soon as tooth eruption starts, regarding initiation of brushing, and a suitable brush may be selected. The avoidance of the presence of food debris in contact with the teeth over long periods and the perils of sticky soothing syrups are emphasized.

As soon as the confidence of the child has been gained and in the vast majority of cases this is on the first visit—a topical fluoride prophylaxis is carried out.

In our practice although many types of fluoride solutions and preparations have been used over the past years, as a matter of standard routine we use 10 per cent stannous fluoride solution (*see* p. 54).

THE EARLY CARIES LESION

At recall the young patient who has had a careful preventive programme will have little or no caries. However sometimes 'sticky' pits or fissures may be detected in recall or new patients. These should not be restored with conventional fillings. The effect of topical stannous fluoride applications should be noted over successive check ups and usually the incipient caries lesion will be found to have become brown and hard. If tempted to prepare a 'prophylactic cavity' the surface of the dentine is often found to be harder than expected (Massler, 1967). These sticky areas have been watched for many years and rarely has a filling been required.

RAMPANT CARIES

The new child patient that presents with rampant caries requires special attention. All too frequently there is a mass of amalgam

a

b

Fig. 34. Rampant caries associated with rose-hip syrups and comforters.

fillings around the mouth with further carious breakdown of these already heavily filled teeth. Cervical decalcifications are frequently seen (*Fig.* 34). Deep carious lesions near, or involving, the pulp may be apparent. No 'permanent' fillings should be placed at this stage.

Treatment should take the following lines:

1. Treat pain by suitable dressings, endodontic techniques, or extractions.

2. Other gross carious lesions are treated by excavating carious dentine and placing dressings usually of the reinforced zinc oxide eugenol type, sometimes with a metacresylacetate dressing sealed over any caries approaching too near the pulp and which has been left in situ.

3. The patient is taught plaque and debris control by careful demonstrations of its effective removal by brushing. A fluoride dentifrice is prescribed.

4. Stannous fluoride topical applications, as described previously.

5. Diet counselling, especially regarding carbohydrate and sucrose, is given to the parent.

6. Shallow cervical decalcifications—crumbly, chalky white areas usually—are treated by careful application of stannous fluoride. They are not 'filled'.

7. The patient is brought back 2–3 weeks after the last dressing is placed, to check brushing ability and plaque control. At this stage a further topical application of stannous fluoride may be carried out.

At the next inspection, i.e. 4 months later, there should be some measure of control of the rampant caries. New cavities rarely will be seen. However, some already existing carious lesions involving deeper layers of dentine may become apparent and these should be treated by excavation and dressings of the reinforced zinc oxide eugenol type.

Treated superficial caries will be seen to darken and harden indicating that remineralization has begun.

Wei et al. (1968) define the remineralization as a replacement of the 'lost calcium and phosphate with other minerals by chemical processes and exchange, substitution and physical and chemical bonding'. They further state that, 'based on radiographic and microradiographic evidence a 10 per cent stannous fluoride solution appears to remineralize carious dentine more rapidly and was superior to other remineralizing solutions'.

As soon as there is a dramatic diminution in new carious lesions permanent restorations may be placed in the 'controlled' mouth. Surface lesions such as the now brown cervical areas may be watched for years, however: eventually some may be restored with 'permanent' materials. Others may be left alone if the discoloration, which fades somewhat in time, is tolerable aesthetically.

It may take 2 years to gain *complete* control of a rampant caries patient but 'immediate' noticeable control is usually effected in

3–4 months. If no caries is discovered for three consecutive check-ups it is permissible to omit the topical 10 per cent stannous fluoride and just gently polish all surfaces with Zircate treatment paste.

Thus it can be seen that prevention of caries at the practice level does not consist merely of applying solutions of fluoride to the teeth. It requires a complete change in attitude and approach on the part of the dentist, the attitude of his patients by parent education, and of his staff which should be organized as a dental health team.

Basic requirements are these:

1. The dentist and his aides must be themselves convinced and confident of the efficacy of a preventive program. Assistants and patients will be influenced by the dentist's enthusiasm.

2. The 'prophylactic odontotomy' approach should be largely abandoned. Fillings and more fillings to prevent fillings does not make sense. There is evidence that the more fillings which patients receive, the more they require. A mouth in which the teeth are peppered with unsightly amalgam fillings on all surfaces has not had the best treatment although many dentists surprisingly consider that they are practising true prevention.

3. The dentist should re-think what constitutes a 'cavity'. Is initial caries attack a 'cavity'? The tendency is to consider that all breaches of surface should be filled. Thus the State dental service actually encourages the filling of 'sticky' pits and fissures, i.e. those teeth where a sharp probe will just 'stick'. This has been conventional teaching and it seems to be current teaching today. In a real preventive program 'sticky' fissures should not be subjected to cavity preparation and filling, but the effect of topical fluoride over a period should be noted.

4. Even in mouths where there are obviously many cavities requiring treatment this should be planned and action taken to minimize further cavity occurrence. Experience demonstrates to us all the futility of filling cavities in the rampant caries mouth. A short time later there is another 'crop' of cavities. The rampant caries mouth is a special situation mouth, which Massler has called the 'caries infected mouth', and he has postulated control of the infection before embarking on extensive restorations (Massler, 1967).

5. The dentist must be careful not to be the causation of dental disease or recurrent disease. This may happen in the following ways:

    a. Inadequate preparations leading to further breakdown of weak enamel walls.

    b. Poor restorations leading to leaking and recurrent caries, and filling overhangs which may be influential in gingival problems.

   c. Over-enthusiastic polishing of teeth with brushes and pumice which scratch the surface and favour plaque attachment.

   d. Over-enthusiastic polishing of fillings which may overheat amalgam and affect its physical properties and also the use of abrasives may tend to lessen resistance to caries attack by removing the protective layer of enamel containing the most fluoride ion.

THE HANDICAPPED CHILD

Special consideration must be given to the handicapped child (or adult), although it should be borne in mind that more often than not the patient will not be as conscious of the handicap as the operator. However, handicapped patients require more time, thought and care in oral hygiene training and many of them will need more efficient plaque removal than their more fortunate contemporaries.

Distressingly there are too many different handicaps to list but we may consider the following categories:

  1. *Heart*   Congenital
                        Rheumatic (acquired)
  2. *Senses*   Blindness
                        Deafness
  3. *Limbs*   Arm movements defective
                        Leg movements defective
  4. *Mental Defects*   Continuous
                        Periodic: Petit mal
                                 Grand mal
  5. *Generalized Systemic Diseases*, e.g. Leukaemia.

     The dental team should evolve their own techniques for dealing with these main categories and should thus be prepared and not have to devise anything but to modify the approach for the individual patient.

1. *Congenital Heart Disease*

Here exceptional oral hygiene control is imperative, with antibiotic cover for all procedures which might provoke bacteriaemia. Increase of antibiotic dosage may be necessary during dentistry for those already on regular maintenance antibiotic therapy.

Rheumatic Heart Disease requires the same considerations as above, and these patients are more likely to be on permanent antibiotic cover. The risk for all these heart patients is, of course, the possibility of bacterial endocarditis. All septic areas (or potentially septic areas) should be removed under suitable chemotherapy cover.

The successful handling of these cases will depend on a careful history, records and a close co-operation with the patient's physician at all times.

2. Senses—Blindness and Deafness

The difficulty which must be overcome in teaching oral care methods, is of course, communication and demonstration.

The *deaf* will benefit by visual aids and carefully written instruction sheets for home reading. An intermediary who uses finger sign language may help to solve their communication problem.

The *blind*. Use of large tactile teaching aids such as models with large tooth brushes will help considerably. Cassette tapes may also be prepared and given for home use.

3. Defective Limb Movements

This calls for assistance of a third party or in lesser handicaps the use of various aids such as automatic brushes, patent floss holders, 'perio aids', may be tried, probably successively until one suitable for the patient is discovered.

4. Mental Handicaps

For those on phenytoin to control epileptic seizures it is essential to teach or somehow to ensure plaque control to avoid the tendency for gross enlargement of the gingivae. There is no doubt that this will not occur in the 100 per cent clean mouth (a difficult, often impossible achievement with anyone, but much more difficult with most epileptics).
5. Careful oral cleansing with as much freedom from trauma as possible is essential with leukaemics, often antibiotic cover is required. No extraction should be carried out without very special precautions being taken and it is better to refer the child to a hospital.

On the whole whatever other handicaps may be mentioned—cleft palate, diabetes, etc.—the main essentials will be the preservation of the teeth, the avoidance of major operative interference and hence primary prevention from the earliest possible moment in order to prevent the onset of destructive disease.

PREVENTIVE ASPECTS OF ORTHODONTICS

Consideration was given to the inclusion of a chapter on interceptive orthodontics by an eminent consultant in this field. It was felt, however, that the experience of someone who looked at the patient from the viewpoint of the general practitioner and who was very conscious of his own limitations with regard to orthodontic procedures would probably enable the reader to 'identify' more easily.

As a general practitioner the author many years ago carried out more orthodontic treatment for patients than in later years. Enthusiasm was dampened by failures which occurred and which were directly due to trying to deal with situations which were beyond one's skill and diagnostic capability. Most of such cases were those in which abnormal skeletal patterns presented. Cases in which there were localized irregularities or crowding responded well to the simple forms of treatment.

a

b

Fig. 35. Retained *A/A* causing malalignment of 1/1.

The dentist must be watchful of his young patients to check from say age 5 onwards the development of the arches and their relationship to each other. The size, shape and quality of the teeth must be taken into account because crowding which involves a genetically determined factor such as large teeth and small arches may involve some difficulty to resolve—it may not be accomplished by appliances,

87

but on the other hand the timing of the dentist's involvement is important because later growth of the jaws may deal with the problem anyway. What the dentist must be careful of is subjecting a child to prolonged periods of appliances and retention devices.

During his regular examinations of the child there should be careful recording of possibly harmful habits such as thumb sucking, tongue thrusting, lip habits, incorrect swallowing patterns, and possibly one could also include mouth breathing. Many of the deformities (such as anterior open bite associated with thumb and finger sucking) will correct themselves in time, if and when the child stops the habit, and therefore the dentist must here too be aware of the timing for interception. Many of these habits, if persisted in, call for much care, tact and ingenuity in therapy and often for considerable co-operation between dentist, parent and the physician.

The careful dentist who has prepared properly articulated study models will soon realize whether he is dealing with a Class II or Class III malrelationship. He would do well to refer these cases to a consultant orthodontist for advice and treatment. No orthodontic treatment should be embarked on without very careful consideration of the total arch relationships. However, the following may well be considered as being within the scope of preventive attention.

1. Retained deciduous teeth. The ankylosed tooth especially may cause malalignment of the permanent tooth and may also cause lack of development of the alveolar process. (*Fig.* 35).

2. Poor restorative attention—loss of contacts due to caries or inadequately contoured fillings may lead to loss of space posteriorly while overcontoured posterior contact areas may cause anterior crowding.

3. Loss of deciduous posterior teeth may lead to encroachment on the space required for eruption of successional teeth. (*Fig.* 36). Attention should be paid to the necessity for provision of a space maintainer but *careful* observation over a period may determine whether this is necessary, which is not always the case.

4. Crossbites in wholly deciduous arches usually do not require orthodontic interference as the permanent arches are not usually corrected by this early treatment.

5. Unerupted or erupted supernumerary teeth may cause mal-alignment (as in (1) above). (*See Fig.* 37).

6. Individual teeth which are in incorrect labiolingual relationship with their opponents may be corrected by simple bite-plane appliances (i.e. they can be moved over the arch by a bite-raiser and inclined plane); once in the correct relationship no retention will be required.

a

b

c

Fig. 36. *a, b,* A marked upper anterior irregularity at age 12 caused by two palatal supernumeraries. *c,* The completed good result.

89

The dentist must always be prepared to take further advice should there be any doubt, and certainly he must be fully conscious of the consequences of the long-term effects of any extractions, whether serial or symmetrical and be especially careful when considering extraction of a crowded anterior tooth.

It is necessary to carry out careful radiographic examination of

a

b

Fig. 37. *a*, Loss of a deciduous tooth with space encroached upon by first molar. *b*, A space maintainer would prevent this.

both jaws in order to record presence or absence of successional teeth and supernumeraries. A panoramic examination is the radiography of choice.

For details of methods and techniques the dentist is referred to one of the many excellent orthodontic texts especially intended for the general practitioner.

REFERENCES

Dickson G. C. (1965) *Orthodontics in General Dental Practice.* London, Pitman.

Geiger A. and Hirschfeld L. (1974) *Minor Tooth Movement in General Practice.* St. Louis, Mosby.

Massler M. (1967) Changing concepts in the treatment of carious lesions. *Br. Dent. J.* **123,** 457.

Tulley W. J. (1967) Prevention in orthodontics within the scope of the school programme. *Int. Dent. J.* **17,** 368–383.

Tulley W. J. and Campbell A. C. (1974) *A Manual of Practical Orthodontics,* 3rd ed. Bristol, Wright.

Walther D. P. (1967) *Orthodontic Notes,* 2nd ed. Bristol, Wright.

Wei S. H. Y., Kaqueler J. C. and Massler M. (1968) Remineralization of carious dentine. *J. Dent. Res.* **47,** 381.

PREVENTIVE ASPECTS OF RESTORATIVE DENTISTRY

CURRENT views on restorative dentistry tend to support the broad general principles of G. V. Black (1908) but with some modifications. The original concept of extension for prevention was to ensure that the prepared cavity margins were placed in self-cleansing areas. In order to conserve tooth structure the preparation of class 2 cavities is extended only into 'cleansable areas', i.e. areas which are accessible to the toothbrush. Thus, in all cavity preparation the modifications are such as to avoid excessive tooth reduction. The ease with which tooth structure can be destroyed since the advent of the air-turbine drill calls for strict discipline and self control in its use.

In preparing proximal cavities it is essential to avoid damage to the contacting neighbouring tooth surface by being touched by the high speed burr. The placing of a metal matrix strip between the teeth during drilling will protect the intact surface, or it can be so arranged that the final break-through of the contact area is made with hand instruments. In restoring the same area it is important for the health of the soft tissues to ensure a naturally restored and well contoured proximal surface with good tight contact with the next tooth. The use of contoured matrix bands with suitably shaped wedges is essential for the above restorative procedures, and this applies not only to amalgam but is even more important in the anterior regions with the currently used composite filling materials which are not only difficult to distinguish from tooth structure but are very troublesome to remove.

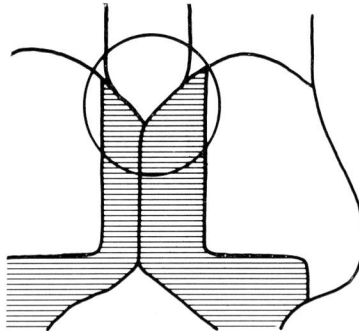

Fig. 38. A flattened contact area encourages food packing. A space opens up fairly rapidly between the teeth because of the wear between the flat surfaces.

A flattened contact area will close up the embrasure, which should normally be triangular in shape, and this will either crowd out any existing papilla, or will prevent accessibility to cleansing, and food will pack in from the occlusal (*Figs.* 38–40).

A well-restored marginal ridge will provide deflecting contours which will protect the interdental area.

If there is difficulty with amalgam in achieving a tight contact with the proximal tooth, consideration must be given to the use of a gold inlay. So far the experience with composite fillings in these situations is that the contacts become worn very rapidly.

It has been noted that occasionally some dentists, on failing to achieve a tight contact will open up the interdental area even more, in the belief that food will 'wash right through'. It is a poor remedy and rarely succeeds because it usually requires a separation of at least half a tooth in width and this amount of space will often result in tooth drift and loss of arch stability.

It is assumed that by now the dentist carrying out restorative procedures will be aware of the necessity of ensuring that the patient has previously been trained in plaque elimination methods. Therefore in crown or inlay construction the trend should be to prepare the margins supragingivally, as far as aesthetics will allow. Although it was taught for generations that in order to avoid recurrent caries the margins should be placed in the gingival sulcus or crevice, the disadvantage of gingival irritation, overhang problems, and possible operative damage to the attachment apparatus indicates avoidance of this situation as far as possible. If caries or other considerations necessitate preparation deep into the crevice care should be taken at the impression stage not to use destructive gingival retraction methods. Astringent cords or rings should be left in place for a few minutes only, and if electrosurgical methods are employed, strict precautions should be taken to avoid soft tissue or bone necrosis.

Much has been written about the importance of deflecting contours on the buccal and lingual surfaces of crowns, and the perils of not reproducing the ideal form. It is probable that there has been some over-statement, but the undercontoured crown with a flat surface may act as a plane for shedding food directly into the gingival crevice, and this may be harmful to the susceptible patient. Far more harmful is, as previously stated, the poorly contoured contact area. The size of artificial crowns and pontics is important, and in general they should be smaller in buccolingual width and in the amount of occlusal area compared to the natural teeth. (*See Fig.* 41.)

Pontics in fixed bridgework should present a 'bullet nose' contact with the alveolar ridge, and the embrasures of the bridgework should be free. The patient should be instructed in daily cleaning, and some will need to be shown the use of floss threaders (such as Zon

a

b

c

Fig. 39. Lack of adequate embrasure spaces has caused the deep pocketing and bone loss (*a*, *b*) The raised periodontal flap (*c*) shows the extent of the damage.

94

Fig. 40. The importance of a good well-contoured matrix band and wedges cannot be overstressed. Many teeth are imperilled by filling overhangs. This one must have been the result of exceptionally over-enthusiatic amalgam packing. The second molar was unsaveable.

Fig. 41. The well-known 'gum-stripper' denture (which is still being made!). The sharp collets are mechanical irritants and the contoured gum fitted edges hold plaque against gingivae and teeth.

or Nupons) in order to introduce the floss under any soldered contact points. The amount of effort and time that the patient will have to expend should be minimal and will depend on the care and thought which has gone into the design and construction of the restoration. The importance of good polishing techniques is described elsewhere.

It should always be remembered that all restorations eventually leak at the margins and therefore there is no such thing as a 'preventive filling'. However, preference should be given to those cements, lining agents, or restorative materials which contain fluorides, as there is evidence that they reduce the incidence of recurrent caries. (This was a notable finding with the fluoride containing silicate fillings.)

REFERENCES

Black G. V. (1908) *Operative Dentistry.* Chicago, Medical & Dental Publishing.

Burch J. G. (1971) Ten rules for developing crown contours in restorations. *Dent. Clin. North Am.* **15,** 611–618.

Marcum J. S. (1967) The effect of crown margin and depth upon gingival tissue. *J. Prosthet. Dent.* **17,** 479–487.

Skurow H. M. and Lytle J. D. (1971) "The interproximal embrasure" *Dent. Clin. North Am.* **15,** 641–647.

Waerhaug J. and Zander H. A. (1957) Reaction of gingival tissues to self-curing acrylic restorations. *J. Am. Dent. Assoc.* **54,** 760.

CHAPTER 8

PREVENTIVE DENTISTRY AND SPORTS ACTIVITIES

INJURIES to the teeth and jaws occur in a variety of sporting activities and games. It should be a responsibility of the dental profession to advise on measures to cut down the rate of occurrence of these injuries and to take steps to protect any of their patients involved in risky sports, to minimize the dangers.

Two kinds of activities may be considered:

1. 'Contact' sports in which physical involvement between players is an essential element. Examples are rugby football, boxing, wrestling, and to a lesser extent soccer.
2. 'Individual' sports which may involve dangers. Examples are cycling, motor racing, cricket, baseball and swimming.

The dentist should determine whether any of his patients are likely to be involved in sporting activities likely to result in trauma to face or jaws and to assess whether any protection can be given.

In the U.S.A. it is mandatory for all schools to ensure that those engaged in contact sports are provided with mouth protectors in games such as American football. There would appear to be considerable controversy regarding the role to be played by dentists in relation to the fitting of mouth protectors, and in fact much of this work is done by the team trainer and is accepted by him as an extra source of income.

At the practice level it has been found that fractured teeth would appear to be associated most frequently with the non-contact sports. This may be due to the fact that with recognized dangerous activities such as boxing and rugby football there are usually facilities for dealing rapidly with injuries of all kinds, and fractured or avulsed teeth or jaw injuries are dealt with by immediate hospital referral. It is also probable that many of the players are already wearing mouth protectors. Fractured teeth have been reported most often from accidents arising in cricket, cycling and swimming. These are activities in which it is not reasonable to expect the wearing of mouth protectors for obvious reasons. The dentists' responsibility here is one of warning of possible dangers.

The provision of mouth protectors where feasible, i.e. in fairly short activities of a combative nature, have been demonstrably successful. The fabrication and design of a mouth protector should of course be considered in the same light as the motor car safety belt.

There should be an organized programme to ensure that the device is worn. Where school activities are involved, encouragement, or even enforcement, should be the responsibility of the school but the dentist should be aware of the problem and check that his patient is not exposed to an avoidable hazard through ignorance or neglect.

Mouth Protectors

They should be comfortable to wear, protect the teeth and the gingivae, and should not affect breathing or speech. Three types of mouth protectors are usually considered: (1) Stock prefabricated vinyl protectors; (2) Protectors with individual modification in the mouth; (3) Individually fabricated mouth protectors (*Fig.* 42).

Most protectors are made for the maxilla.

1. The stock mouth protector is usually supplied in three different sizes: small, medium and large. The appropriate size is chosen for each person and trimmed as necessary to fit on the upper jaw. Some remoulding in the mouth is possible by prior immersion in hot water. These protectors are generally considered to be unsatisfactory because they are loose and thus are not well tolerated. Also there would not necessarily be proper coverage of vulnerable areas.

2. Mouth formed protectors. These are usually supplied in a kit containing a plastic shell, often vinyl, which is matched to the upper arch and trimmed where necessary. The fitting surface is filled with a mixed soft acrylic or silicone and put to place on the maxillary teeth where the material is allowed to set while the teeth are gently closed together. Further trimming of the margins is carried out.

Disadvantages are the necessary excess bulk and therefore lack of comfort and interference with speech. The device is not easy to adjust for occlusion and therefore the wearer tends to chew through or tear it.

This method of protection is, however, reasonably quick and is less expensive than the custom-made protectors. One side-advantage is the possible use of these for fluoride application by filling the tooth side with phosphate fluoride gel and allowing the wearer to chew for four minutes. (This is of course of added benefit compared with those protectors less carefully adapted and which therefore can be reversed for either jaw, i.e. with the stock protectors.)

3. The protector made by a dental technician or a dental auxiliary to individual models is to be preferred. Stronger material—usually vinyl blanks—can be vacuum formed.

Advantages are careful coverage of vulnerable areas, lack of excessive bulk and the care which can be taken not to encroach too much on the free way space occlusally.

a

b

Fig. 42. Mouth protectors which may be remoulded and trimmed to fit the individual. Note the plastic bag for storing protector between games.

99

The protection of teeth and jaws, where possible by the use of mouth protectors, is a good exercise for the combined efforts of the dental team—in communication, advice and technique of fabrication. The hygienist should instruct in the care of the protector—careful cleaning after use and storage in a clean container.

Dentists who treat patients who have special athletic distinction and who are likely to compete for honours in such gatherings as the Olympic Games must be aware that these patients may require special care. Often these athletes travel to distant countries and many cases have been cited where dental emergencies have interfered with, or cancelled, the athlete's performance. It is not sufficient merely to check for caries. A complete radiographic examination should be done (ideally with panoramic radiography), and the gingival condition should be evaluated. It is of the utmost importance to pay particular attention to the problem of partly erupted third molars. In these patients, third molar periocoronitis would appear to be the main cause of emergencies and hence all doubtful third molars should be removed well before an important contest.

REFERENCES

Bureau of Dental Health Education and Bureau of Economic Research and Statistics (1964) Evaluation of mouth protectors used by high school football players. *J. Am. Dent. Assoc.* **68**, 430.

Forrest J. O. (1969) The dental condition of Olympic Games contestants—a pilot study. *Dent. Pract. Dent. Rec.* **20**, 95.

Godwin W. C. and Craig R. G. (1968) Stress transmitted through mouth protectors *J. Am. Dent. Assoc.* **77**, 1316–1320.

Hertz W. D. (1968) Mouth protectors: a progress report. *J. Am. Dent. Assoc.* **77**, 632.

Stenger J. M., Lawson E. A., Wright J. M. et al. (1964) Mouthguards: protection against shock to head neck and teeth. *J. Am. Dent. Assoc.* **69**, 273.

APPENDIX 1

MATERIALS FOR USE IN THE PREVENTIVE PRACTICE

R = Recommended.

Demonstration Models and Teaching Materials
(For toothbrushing instruction and explanation of the structure of the teeth and supporting tissues.)
  Information regarding these may be obtained from the Oral Hygiene Service, Hesketh House, Portman Square, London W1. Other audio-visual aids may be obtained from Messrs Nesor, London.

Toothbrushes

R　Wisdom Multituft (0·011 in filaments) (Medium)
　Oral B 40　　　　(0·007 in filaments)
　Oral B 30　　　　(0·007 in filaments) for the small mouth
　Gibbs Short head　(0·009 in filaments)
　Automatic Toothbrushes:　Ronson (rechargeable only);
　　　　　　　　　　　　　　Broxodent (mains);
　　　　　　　　　　　　　　Phillips (rechargeable only).

Floss

Waxed (Johnson & Johnson).
Unwaxed (Johnson & Johnson, if available).
'Dentotape' (Johnson & Johnson, if available). This is still probably the most acceptable floss. It is hoped that it will be available in the U.K. in the near future. Other makes of floss, nearly all imported from the U.S.A., are available at the dental depots. In spite of considerable pressure in favour of unwaxed floss there is little clinical evidence to suggest that its practical difficulties in use are compensated by any degree of superiority over conventional waxed floss.

Interdental Cleansers and 'Stimulators': Wooden Sticks

R　1.　Stimudents (from U.S.A.).
　　2.　Inter-dens (local pharmacy).
R　3.　Sanodents (obtainable in U.K. from Boots Chemists only).
　　4.　Jordan's Interdental Sticks.

101

Interdental Brushes and Tips

R   Interspace brush (Halex).
Jordan Interdental Brush.
Perio-pak (Crescent).
Perio-aid (Butler).

Disclosing Solutions and Devices

R   *'Displaque'* (Pacemaker; Dental suppliers).
'Disclosing Wafers' Procter & Gamble.
'Ceplac' *Disclosing tablets* (Local pharmacy).
Rosepink food dye (Rayners; Food shops or Rayners, London).
Red Cote (Solution only) (Butler; Dental suppliers).
C Red solution (En De Kay; S. S. White).
Plaklite Electrical apparatus using fluorescein dye. (*see text*). Should be available shortly in U.K.
Iodine-based solution (Iodine: 1·6 g KI: 1·6 g Water: 13·4 ml Glycerine to make 30 ml.

Water Jet Irrigation Devices

Water Pik This is no longer on the accepted list of the Council on Dental Therapeutics of the American Dental Association (*see* pp. 25–6).

Fluorides

For Topical Application

R   1. Stannous fluoride topical kit. Messrs Procter & Gamble, Caulk.
2. Hi Fluor APF solution and gels. (Dental Science Advancement Foundation, or Allied Laboratories.)
3. Various topical fluoride gels and solutions from the dental supply houses, e.g. from S. S. White (En De Kay).
4. Applicator trays for APF gels. Various makes, e.g. Fluotray (En De Kay), Pascal, Hi Fluor.

Fluoride Prophylaxis Pastes

R   Zircate treatment paste (with stannous fluoride). (Caulk.)
Fluoride prophylaxis paste (En De Kay).

Systemic and Local Fluoride Ingestion

Fluoraday lac tablets. 2·2 mg NaF. (Dental Health Promotion.)
Fluotabs. En De Kay. 2·2 mg NaF. (S. S. White.)
Fluodrops. En De Kay. 1·1 mg NaF in 0·3 ml = 10 drops (S. S. White).
(Preferable for infants under 2 years of age.)

102

Fluoride Rinses

Combined 0·4 per cent stable stannous fluoride and APF (Janar Inc., U.S.A., when available.)

Fluoride Dentifrices

Acceptable from Colgate, Beechams, Procter & Gamble, Elida-Gibbs, or other manufacturers of similar repute.

Desensitizing Dentifrices

For sensitive necks of teeth.

Emoform   } Europe
Thermodent } U.S.A.
Sensodyne

These dentifrices are *not* intended for sore or inflamed gingivae. They should not be used for any soft tissue lesion.

Mouthwashes for General Use

R   Warm Water.

R   Normal Saline. 1·0 per cent NaCl in water.

Mouthwashes other than saline solution or warm water are rarely required and the use of peroxyborate solutions is likely on balance to do more harm than good.

Polishing Materials for use by the Dentist or Hygienist

For finishing and polishing restorations, and polishing the teeth after prophylaxis.

Contra-angle polishing head—snap-on or screw-in.
Small cup bristle brushes—snap-on or screw-in.
Rubber polishing cups—snap-on or screw-in.
Small rubber polishing wheels, screw mandrel.
Green and red rubber polishing cones—mounted.
Moyco coarse—medium 4 mm cuttle strips.
Moyco extra-fine—narrow 2·5 mm cuttle strips.
3M composite polishing strips, fine/medium.
3M composite discs 2 grits, fine/medium.
Zirconium silicate powder or paste.
Zirconium silicate and stannous fluoride paste.
Finishing burrs—blunt, round and flame-shaped.
blunt, friction grip tapered fissure, carbide burrs.

SUMMARY OF PROCEDURE FOR PREVENTION OF CARIES AND PERIODONTAL DISEASE

THIS is essentially the procedure carried out to ensure that disease does not occur rather than the more usual treatment of already established disease, i.e. the causes are dealt with rather than the effects.

The dentist knows and makes the patient aware that plaque is very considerably involved in the causation of caries and periodontal disease.

The dentist explains to the patient the change of attitude from repair to prevention. This is related to the patient's present condition and past history of repeated or progressive disease.

The preventive methods advocated for the patient are outlined.

The hygienist may take over at the next stage and may carry out a series of preventive sessions during which the patient's plaque control ability is assessed and the patient is trained in the effective use of the toothbrush, possible use of dental floss and visits are continued until the patient can successfully perform the methods taught (usually 4 to 5 visits).

It must be emphasized that if we have to choose the most important single change which exemplifies today's preventive approach, it would not be plaque control methods, or fluoridation. It would be the realization that drilling a tooth is never a preventive measure but always a repair. Therefore cutting cavities must be done only when unavoidable, and when the previously described preparation has been completed.

The Child

Up to age 10. The mother or responsible adult should be taught the care of the child's mouth—with the child as interested listener. Topical fluorides are applied on a 4-monthly basis and a fluoride dentifrice is recommended.

1. Regular 4-monthly checks and prophylaxis after the patient has been rendered dentally healthy and is fully co-operating with oral hygiene.

2. At intervals of one year there should be a complete reappraisal and retraining if necessary in plaque control—brushing, floss, etc.

3. It is customary in the U.K. to take 2 radiographs as caries check at roughly yearly intervals. Over the years this is *entirely inadequate* for complete diagnostic procedures, and for patients 'at risk'—through caries or periodontal disease—a full mouth study should be considered about every 3 years. A better alternative is a panoramic study (OPG—orthopantomograph or Panorex).

The current situation and the progress over the years—deterioration, improvement or static condition—should be discussed, with advice as to whether there should be changes made in the light of the new information.

After this the child or adolescent is taught separately but the parent may be called in to reinforce training at any stage. The parent is especially involved, however, in discussion of diet and the effects of sucrose, together with advice such as avoiding consuming sugary substances, but if sweets are given they should be associated with a mealtime and not throughout the day.

The use of topical anticaries agents is discussed with the parent and arrangements are made to make these applications every school holiday. Parents may be informed (depending on the dentist's arrangements) that the parents' responsibility will be to remember that school holiday means 'visit to the dentist', and therefore there will not be any recalls made.

A recommendation as to the type of toothbrush is made and an accepted fluoride dentifrice may be presented.

One great fallacy which seems to be repeated in all preventive dentistry texts is to consider the preventive approach in relation to *new* patients. The patient in danger is the regularly attending patient —year after year with never a really complete examination and assessment after the first one. It is too easy to become complacent about the regularly attending patient. The intervention of a third party, e.g. another dentist or hygienist with a fresh questioning eye, may often provide evidence and a warning that all is not well with the patient. There should therefore be a long-term care plan worked out for each patient with a programme such as previously outlined.

All 'old' patients require regular re-evaluation—new history, new thorough examination, especially for the presence of gingival pockets and mobility or drifting of teeth. Treatment should be formulated and revised if necessary, taking into account the patient's tissue response and attitude to dental care.

SOME PRACTICAL PROBLEMS

AN extraordinary amount of physical change may often occur. Dietary habits may be altered—e.g. there are periods of lemon addiction with some patients, often associated with enamel erosion, or a previously heavy smoker gives up and perhaps starts to suck sugary mint tablets and a crop of cervical caries may result. An ageing patient may suffer from dry mouth, again with a greater tendency to caries. Thus the importance of constant vigilance with one's current patients is to be stressed.

In spite of careful preventive attention some patients will develop carious cavities. It is important, therefore never to promise '100 per cent freedom from the drill' a phrase often used by newspapers. Similarly we are unable to promise that periodontal disease will never occur. But our methods *will* diminish the incidence of these diseases to manageable proportions. We should not, therefore, have a sense of guilt because of the discovery of the occasional cavity or incipient periodontal lesion as long as patients have had all the care and vigilance which our preventive approach demands.

We must not accept an accusation of failure on these occasions from our patients. This can be avoided by previously telling them that we cannot promise total absence of disease.

An awkward situation may occur when one of our long-term preventive patients attends another practice for some reason (perhaps because of a move from the district). If the dentist is similarly enthusiastic about prevention all will be well. Sometimes, however, the new dentist belongs to the school of 'pit and fissure haters', who feel that all virgin pits and fissures ought to be drilled out if they are 'sticky'. (We might have been watching these 'sticky' fissures for years without deterioration in them.) The patient may be told that he or she *needs*, say, 6 fillings. The patient becomes understandably indignant at what is alleged to be the failure of our prevention. We have such patients who have received six or more tiny amalgam fillings barely into the dentine. It is necessary therefore to warn patients that such a situation may arise, and if there is any doubt to ask for a second opinion.

INDEX